YOGA
FOR
EVERYONE

RECONCILE YOUR SOUL

"YOGA IS THE JOURNEY
of the self,
THROUGH THE SELF,
TO THE SELF "
- THE BHAGAVAD GITA

Dedicated to all yoga practitioners

<u>DISCLAIMER</u>

Author : Sanjeev Thakur

For more informations,questions,comments and requests regarding yoga educational material,consulations,programs you are welcomed and should be addressed to:

Hno.4 Upper Vishnulok ,Tapovan
Dehradun,Uttarakhand,India
Website – www.yogaanart.com
email – infoworldcreations@gmail.com
Mob – +91-9760438992

Yoga Conscience

- Moral rationality of the soul

Yoga is an art. A way of living. It originates from our Conscience that heals our body mind and soul in a spiritual way. We can say that yoga is the food of the Soul. The food or diet we consume for our daily physical activities but for the soul the food is the yoga that involves breathing, asanas, meditation, several kriyas with proper discipline.

It is the proven fact that the roots of yoga are inherited in our Conscience. The will or resolute should be to motivate self to grow the roots continuously in an unconscious manner and to transform the roots into a huge tree that that will flower our life so that it may be fruitful to all of us. The life will be blissful and prosperous in wisdom.

Conscience is the moral rationality of the soul. Yoga is the action process derived from our Conscience where it is deep rooted. Then it becomes a natural phenomenon of action in everything we do and perform. This routine is similar to our breathing system that happens in a subconscious manner without putting any effort.

This is the Conscience that heals us in a subconscious way that motivates us constantly in our every actions that makes us believe that missing yoga sometimes makes us uneasy and interference in gaining of the divine energy.

Yoga Conscience is the art of liberation from our desires and to constantly grow our energy level. It is the belief in our moral values. The increase level in our self confidence. It makes us strong. The inherent belief that we can overcome all obstacles and hindrance in whatever we face or get surrounded with. The hope of non illness, healthy and fit .The increase of immunity and will to win. The growth in our energy level.

Conscience and life are interrelated deeply. A new born baby shows the glimpse of his presence in one or the other way. For the adults conscience take birth in other form. He acts according to the situation. Conscience is itself a form of awakening unknowingly or reaction according to situation and surroundings.

If we look at history we will find so many great ideals that have left their signs of greatness facing and fighting immense obstacles and problems but they have never left the fire of their Conscience. These great people were not only their country ideals but the light bearer for the entire society and mankind.

The belief cannot be negated that the Conscience general basics is connected to Indian mythology and the Vedas. We can thus understand the Conscience in Vedic, Dharmic or religious, cultural concept only. Yoga is born from this concept of Conscience.

When in our daily routines we see or hear any inhuman act, our state of mind screams. We feel frustrated, pathetic and agonized. Any indifference or such sinful act by the evil doer means his senses is lost. He cannot differentiate between right or wrong. His Conscience is dead.

Actually in our lifespan we define good or the bad to the level of our Conscience. This is the Conscience we develop the thinking process or mechanics that gives birth to wishes and feelings. Often feelings subdue our thinking process. Knowingly in control to wishes we are trapped to our feelings and then we try to escape from right thinking. In order to not to face this we should always try to scratch the right Conscience. Spiritual knowledge is effective in this scenario. Although it is possible only by awakening of our Conscience.

Yoga Conscience is beyond our mind. While mind behaves in a rational way for our decision process or thought process but Conscience is the self guidance of rightness or wrongness of the thought process. The awareness of our action to do right.

So Yoga should not be confined to just poses and exercises alone but the Conscience is the motivation of its holistic benefits to our overall well being and not only to gain physical benefits but also spiritual awakening to become a liberated soul.

Yoga Conscience is the effort of fulfillment that we always struggled for to live in peace, to live in silence, to be within ourselves, to discover our trueness and be our own masters.

ALTHOUGH THIS BOOK PRIMARY COVERS TOPICS RELATED TO YOGA AND ITS BENEFITS BUT I SHOULD QUOTE THE FOLLOWING LINES OF SWAMI VIVEKANANDA THAT I ALWAYS FOLLOWED WITH YOGA –

" Purity,patience,perseverance
and above all love are the three essentials to success.
Great occasions rouse even the lowest of human beings
to some kind of greatness,
but he alone is the great whose character is great,always."

Table of Contents

Yoga as a way of life

Yoga as a way of life that is elaborate and can easily roundup as a comprehensive workout for a person.Yoga develops positive effects and have an impact on personal, psychological, and spiritual well-being.For anyone who is blessed with yoga, knows deeply how yoga art can have life-changing effects for one's psyche.You will just come to understand yoga as a way of life and recognize its true essence.

Yoga is definitely beyond any set of poses that improve a person's flexibility while improving posture.

Yoga corelates various physical, mental and spiritual activities.These activities help in improving a person's health standards. These are not just exercises. They are considered to be the source code for leading a healthy life.This is something that helps to create a link between individual consciousness and divine consciousness.

There are some forms of yoga that one should be aware of. Some of the most powerful yoga asanas are discussed here. A very famous yoga asana is "Anulom Vilom". This asana helps improve respiratory system performance. In this asana, the physician needs to inhale oxygen from one nostril and exhale from the other. Now, we have to do the same task from the second nostril.

Let us consider Ashtanga yoga for an example.Ashtanga yoga is an ancient practice that focuses on cleansing and purifying the body. This is achieved by synchronized body breath and movement.Ashtanga yoga tones the nervous system and also inspires spiritual enlightenment over time.

In the same way, Iyengar Yoga has been brought into practice by the living guru, BKS. Iyengar.It focuses deeply on the art and science of asana and pranayama.Strength, coordination,an improved flexibility and increased sense of well-being are some of the major benefits of Iyengar yoga.

Pranayama: a way to achieve higher states of awareness.A very interesting word related to yoga is pranayama. Let us know more about the same.Prana refers to vital energy within our body. This is the life force within us. Ayama means control.So Pranayama is the control of breathing.

Through pranayama one can control the pranic energy within the body. This ensures that one has a healthy body and mind. The great yoga guru, Patanjali, referred to pranayama to achieve higher states of awareness. First of all, yoga is a great option for inner peace. With pranayams one can feel inner peace which essentially translates to breathing technique and control.Regulation of air in our body increases metabolism in our system as well as oxygen, which keeps us fresh and energetic.

Kapalabhati: An implementation of Pranayama.Kapalabhati is a yoga technique and a type of pranayama. It initially sounds like a breathing technique, but in short, Kapalbhati has a deeper meaning.

The technique was invented thousands of years ago by Indian yogis. It is believed to be a way of achieving full body fitness. Numerous patients have benefitted greatly by making Kapalbhati a part of their everyday lives.

Benefits of Surya Namaskar

Let us discuss another important word related to yoga, which is Surya Namaskar or Surya Namaskar.Surya Namaskar is an activity performed in the morning at sunrise. It is a compilation of twelve lines, with each pose flowing smoothly to the next section.

Surya Namaskar can be done at a fast pace, or it can be done slowly.A unique feature of Surya Namaskar is that it is a complete workout for the body. While it consists of only 12 sets of exercises, Surya Namaskar has become 288 powerful yoga poses. It occurs over a period of 12 to 15 minutes.

In one round, Surya Namaskar burns around 13.90 calories. Slowly and slowly, you can increase the rounds of Surya Namaskar to 108.

If performed at a slow pace, Surya Namaskar tones the muscles and makes them stronger. Alternatively, Surya Namaskar brings the mind, body and breath in harmony and facilitates a complete meditation experience.

More benefits of yoga

• Then there are several poses to try. They aim to increase your flexibility and balance.

• They also target core muscles and make them stronger.

• Yoga is also very good for weight loss and pain relief.

• Since it moves slowly, there is not much stress on the body to perform and maintain.

• One can do them at a steady pace and aim for perfection of each pose for best results.

• If you are highly ambitious and have a fit body that is used to working, you can try Surya Namaskar. It is a combination of 10 poses, with alternate breathing and breathing patterns for each pose. Needless to say, it targets every part of your body and it can be effective.

Yoga as a way of life is a very wide field and is not limited to physical activities only. There are many meditation poses that help bring the right balance in your life. Due to stress and anxiety, there are examples of which a person is suffering from various diseases due to these. To deal with these problems, you need to do yoga asanas.

Lotus posture is very effective for dealing with stress and anxiety.In this, the practitioner needs to sit with bent legs and has to breathe vigorously. It helps in improving the blood flow in the body and relieving stress.

Due to the many benefits associated with it, more and more people are introducing yoga in their daily lives. It also increases the demand for certified yoga instructors. There are many yoga schools which are offering various courses in which enthusiasts learn various forms of asana and pranayama. You should join these courses to learn this ancient science in a comprehensive way.

As you build proximity to nature, you come to know that it is natural resources that hold the key to eternal health and well-being and making yoga as a way of life.

The Law of energy flow in Yoga

The law of energy

Energy is eternal and all around that grows within us when we arouse it by following yoga practices.Yoga ignites this energy that is divine and blissful that surround us or grasp us internally and externally.The source of this energy is regular flow of pran yoga within us.This is the energy we are searching for that is flowing freely and vibrantly by doing yoga practices that involves breathing,asanas,meditation.Self awareness,discipline and right guidance is strictly observed in all these yoga practices that literally becomes a habit in all our actions and deeds that we do.

What is that energy that grows slowly and steadily that we feel and are regularly motivated to grow that blissful energy? Yes,certainly there is a law of energy a yogi should know and feel and practice to gain or grow that eternal energy slowly and steadily that is the very base of yoga.In fact we can say it as root of yoga.Physical exercise,asanas,mudras are all subsidiary to gain the real resource or energy.

Basic direction of energy movement

Food – Energy gain

Sleep – Energy maintained / Stored

Awakening – Energy released

Pranayama – Energy is Awakened

Pledge / Dhaarna – Energy is focused

Meditation / Dhyan –Movement of energy upwards

Fear – Energy shrinks

Desire - Movement of energy downwards

Love- Flow of energy everywhere that is elaborate and extensive

Samadhi – Energy combines with the divine being.Merge with the universe.

Let us discuss above factors in detail

Food – The food or diet that we intake daily to perform our daily activities is the source of energy we gain.The food should be satvic and pure.Satvic food removes toxins from our body and prevent us from many ailments.

Sleep – A good sleep make us afresh and energetic.Energy is maintained or restored in the cycle of sleeping.Sleeping time frame should make us relax and energetic to perform our daily activities.Sleep disorders causes various problems and depletion of energy level that is a negative for energy growth.

Awakening – Awakening is a process of regular growing,knowing us inherently,to conquer desires and limitations,rising above senses.it is a continous process of being in our horizon to be awake in all our minute activities.A process of vigilness and alertness to our divine existence.In the process of awakening energy is released.

Pranayama – Pranayama or breathing is very beneficial to us.In this state the energy is awakened or aroused.pranayama should be done regularly.Morning time is the best for that.Anulom vilom or alternate nostril breathing should be done with same preference as breathing.Breathing regenerates our cells thus healing the body.

Dhaarana / Pledge – This is the state when energy is focused due to concentration and cultivation of inner sensory activities or awareness.

Dhyan / Meditation – Dhyan or meditation on the divine is an ultimate source of energy moving upwards.This is the state of blissness.

Fear – A yoga practioner should not fear from unknown.In fact yoga practices removes fear and anxiety. Energy shrinks here.

Desire – Our desires prone us to worldly pleasures and attractions that causes diverting our attention towards unwanted things and unnecessary needs.This consumes our lot of energy.This results in movement of energy downwards.We should practice to control or limit our desires that always grows with each desire fulfilled and becomes a never ending process.

Love – Love is a universal divine phenomena that bounds us to nature and mankind.It is a sense of responsibility and devotion to each creature created by the supreme.Here flow of energy is elaborate and extensive thus healing self and society.

Samadhi – Samadhi is the ultimate stage of energy flow that combines with the divine being and merge with the universe.

We have discussed the law of energy which every yogi or yoga practioners should know and understand and try to aim to gain that energy levels before following yoga journey.

Common yoga practice tips

Specific yoga asanas assist to realign the joints, increase flexibility, restore normal range of motion, and improve overall posture.Asanas also indirectly balance the nervous, cardiovascular, respiratory, endocrine, and digestive systems.The systems in the body work as a symbiotic unit, where a positive change in one system usually results in a complimentary change in all the other systems.On the other hand, if asanas are incorrectly practiced, serious complications may result in the systems mentioned above.

AGE LIMITATIONS: Asanas may be practiced by all age groups, male and female.

AWARENESS: Do not practice the yoga asanas mechanically, be aware of your mental and physical state throughout the practice.

CLOTHING: Wear loose, light, non-binding, comfortable clothing; and remove any jewellery, or constricting accessories that may restrict the blood circulation when practicing yoga as the body must bend, twist or move.

CONTRA-INDICATIONS: Avoid yoga practice if you are: experiencing fractured bones, suffering from an acute or chronic ailment or disease, or recuperating from an operation.Consult a primary health care practitioner before commencing asana practice.

CONSULTATION: It is advisable to consult your physician before embarking on the journey of yoga.Find out if your body is physically fit to endure all the asanas.

DIET: There are no special dietary rules for asana practitioners although it is healthier to eat natural fresh foods in moderation.Eat foods that digest and assimilate easily and make the body feel energetic.

DISTRACTIONS: Mute the cellular or telephone during asana practice.It is also helpful to silence the thoughts.

EMPTY STOMACH: Practice at least 2 or 3 hours after consuming food to ensure the stomach is empty.This is one reason why early dawn or dusk practice is recommended.

EMPTYING THE BOWELS: It is helpful to empty the bowels and bladder before commencing the asanas.

FLUID REPLACEMENT: It is very important to drink lot of during, and after yoga practice.

Drink small sips of water at room temperature.

LIMITS: Recognize the limits of the body's normal range of motion, do not overstretch or force yourself into any asana; do not exceed the body's capacity.

MAT :The mat prevents the feet, hands, and elbows from slipping and sliding.

The contact friction provided by the mat helps the body stretch further without straining to hold slipping limbs.

The yoga mat can easily be rolled and/or folded for use in various asanas, for travel, or to simply carry to yoga class.

MAT MAINTENANCE: The yoga mat is best maintained by wiping it by hand with a soft cloth with vinegar or mild detergent and warm water.

Top loading washing machines should NOT be used to clean the mat, the mat can be damaged during the spin cycle.

Front loading washing machines may be used if the mat becomes very soiled.

MIRROR: If possible, practice under the direct supervision of a professional teacher, if this is not possible, practice in front of a mirror to maintain proper body positioning.

Be aware of proper joint alignment, especially in the ankle, knee, shoulder, and neck regions.

NO STRAINING: Do not exert undue force or overstretch while practicing asanas.

Beginners may find the muscles stiff at first, but after several weeks of regular practice the muscles become very supple.

PAIN: The yoga routine should be pain free.If any unusual pain or discomfort is felt, please stop and consult a professional.

PLACE OF PRACTICE: Practice in a well-ventilated room where it is calm and quiet.Asanas may also be practiced outdoors in a pleasant surroundings around nature.Do not practice in a strong wind, in the cold, in the direct sun, around polluted air, or near unpleasant odors.

Do not practice in the vicinity of furniture or anything that prevents free fall to the ground, especially while performing inversion asanas.Often accidents occur because of falls against an object.

PREGNANCY: Prenatal Yoga is a perfect time to nourish and positively influence a growing foetus.In the 9 months in the womb followed by the 3 subsequent years with the mother, the child establishes fundamental rhythm, thought, breathing patterns, and a core value system

After this period, the child becomes a product of its ever-changing environment.The sitting asanas is helpful during pregnancy as they stretch open the pelvis, making the delivery process easier.The standing asanas strengthen the legs and thighs, and assist to carry the baby in the womb.

The core and Mula Bandha locks are paramount to practice throughout the day during early pregnancy.

These locks are helpful in recognizing and releasing tension in the pelvic muscles.During labor this practice also helps to relax between contractions and prevent fatigue.During pregnancy, the body produces the hormone 'relaxin' which increases flexibility in the ligaments and joints.

Many asanas become easier to practice as the pregnancy progresses.

RELAXATION:REST: After every 2 – 3 asana sequence.This not only rests the body, but also develops awareness of the internal energy patterns, and the mental and emotional processes.

This rest period is as important as the asanas themselves and should not be neglected.

SEQUENCE OF YOGA ASANAS: In the Yoga Series, it is very important that the asanas be practiced in the order described.They are designed in a sequential pattern for a specific reason where one asana leads and prepares the body for the next without causing any injury.

SUNBATHING: Never practice asanas for extended periods under the direct sun or after a long period of sunbathing as the body temperature is overheated.

SWEATING:Use a towel to wipe the sweat dry and change into dry clothing before the relaxation asanas to prevent a chill.

TIME OF PRACTICE: Asanas may be practiced at any time of the day, except after meals.

The activities of digestion have stopped, the mind has no deep impressions on the conscious level, and is relatively empty of thoughts at this time.

Although the muscles are more stiff early in the morning compared to late afternoon, nevertheless, this time has a unique awakening and refreshing experience.

A lemonade drink with sugar and salt is very refreshing and balances the metabolites well.

FREQUENCY: Practice yoga daily, if possible, but no less than three times a week.

Practicing yoga daily is like feeding nutritious food to the body and the mind daily.

The ultimate benefit of yoga arrives when yoga becomes a daily habit in taking care of the body and mind.

As the frequency of practice increases, the mind benefits from stress relief, and the body becomes stronger, more flexible, energetic, and balanced.

How Yoga Changes your Brain

Among the foremost common misconceptions about yoga is that it's just another sort of exercise. Perhaps this is often because people often see yogis stretching and doing pretzel-like poses. However, the truth is that the advantages of yoga are more encompassing than simply the physical. And, thanks to modern technology and functional MRI scans, we're now able to see how regular practice affects your brain.

Here are a number of the mental benefits of yoga and the way it produces those effects by changing the structure of your brain.

Our brains are primarily made from two sorts of tissues: white and grey matter. A normal human brain consists of about 60% substantia alba and 40% grey matter . Both of which play important roles in healthy cognitive functioning, however, each brain tissue type features a different function:

Gray matter consists of your brain cells or neurons. While it's called gray matter, in reality, it is pink in color. That's because while you're alive, blood continuously flows through it. After you die, it turns gray. Due to its concentration of neurons, grey matter is liable for many of your brain's functions, including learning skills and memory. It is also responsible for the functionality of interpreting your senses of sight, hearing, smell, and touch. Additionally, it affects your muscle control and self-awareness.

White matter, on the other hand, are the connections that extend from your brain cells. Its job is to connect different sections of your brain, much like how the internet interconnects the world, by allowing areas of your brain to send and receive signals to one another. As such, healthy substantia alba allows your brain to coordinate your thoughts also as your movements.

In general, both gray and substantia alba complement each other to permit you to think, coordinate movement, and interpret the planet surrounding you.Damage or reduction in one or the opposite area affects your cognitive abilities. How yoga has relevancy to our brain matter is that recent research has shown that yoga increases grey matter volume within the hippocampus and frontal sections of your brain. Research involving a comprehensive study of structural brain scans found that a person's general intelligence is related to the quantity of grey matter therein specific area of the brain. Essentially, the thicker the volume of the gray matter in a region of your brain, the more cells are present there and thus, the more likely to perform better.

Get emotional Freedom through Yoga

Many say that by controlling our thoughts we can control our emotions and behaviors.Some are focusing on body-based solutions — like yoga or exercise to help change behaviors.

Strengthening willpower, getting rid of limiting beliefs or defining our values often popped up in the research too.Confusingly, there is a grain of truth in every bit.

Value-based goals strengthen our motivation and yoga practice can have a great impact.What transforms our behaviors is looking at the entirety of ourselves, in.So 'to harness the power to choose our response', first and foremost, we should look into the need that lies between Stimulus and Response.

In the simplest sense, once we are triggered (by Stimuli), we are out of balance and our thoughts, emotions, body is working with everything it's got to restore the balance.This could be a need for safety, connection, recognition or many others.

Our emotions are often the first to recognize the threats and mobilize us to action even before our thinking kicks in.For example, when we jump out of the way from the speeding car, intellectual involvement is limited because of neocortex, even though highly sophisticated, is slow.And if you think you have power over body think again.

We can become anxious just due to simple dehydration or have lack of empathy when we are in high stress.Our mind, body, and emotions form those responses that do not operate in a vacuum.Instead, it pulls together all the resources it can get its hands on.

They will take into account the facts of the present, experiences and learnings of the past to consider the most appropriate response.Our beliefs about self and our cultural norms, past traumas and unhealthy behaviors, our character attributes and other aspects will also influence the response.

Challenging our beliefs about what makes us happy can be highly impactful too.We feel much more empowered, interested, joyful and determined when we chase goals we care about, not the ones given to us by our family, friends or broader society.

If you tend to think back, then looking into your thoughts could be useful.

Maybe at some point expecting the worst was helpful — for example, helped you get through rejections.

Untangling some of those thought patterns could help you change your behaviors better.

When the weather and seasons modification, we frequently feel our bodies respond.

When it's colder outside, we feel more contained and stiff.When it's warmer, we feel open and supple.

Our hearts are the emotional center of love, joy, gratitude, and peace.However, when we suppress our emotions, they often get stuck down in the hips.we} head to our yoga mat- we feel it.Here are two poses the styles of yoga. you can try to get yourself emotionally free today.Here, we will open the hips and the heart together.Grasp the benefits of yoga.

Start by tucking your left leg underneath your right so the knees are squeezed tightly together in front of you.If this is uncomfortable, simply cross your legs or stack your hips up on a bolster.

Root your sitting bones down into the ground and then reach your right arm up and left your arm back.Reach for the hands behind you or clasp onto your belt for assistance.

Take 5 deep breaths here and then fold forward and hold for another 5-10 breaths.

Slowly unharness and either move on to ensuing cause or follow the opposite facet.

Restorative Pigeon Pose / Eka Pada Raja Kapotasana

Transitioning from Gomukhasana, swing the right leg back and shift the hips so they are square to the front.Make sure the front leg is externally rotated so the knee points toward the front left corner of your mat.

For a deep, supportive variation, place a bolster underneath your hips and one in front of you.Straighten out your back leg and lengthen your spine on an inhale.Drape your torso and head over the bolster and give it a nice hug.Exhale all of your stress and old, toxic thoughts and negative emotions away.

Allow yourself to sink and surrender into this supported pigeon pose.If you need a a lot of dynamic follow of columbiform bird cause, strive the complete variation.You can still use a bolster for support under the hips if needed.

Set the legs up in the same position.This time, keep the torso upright and reach back for your right foot with your right hand.Rotate the arm so that you point the elbow up to the sky and bring the foot closer to your head, eventually reaching back with the other arm.

The importance of Postures in Yoga

Posture is basically the way the body mechanically aligns and positions itself in space throughout the day. Body posture changes each moment in adaptation to numerous activities and stresses.The total visual posture is therefore the long-term average of the total alignment in space. Postural habits developed over the years often reflect the unconscious patterns of the mind. Yoga could be a observe that may bring the body back to optimum posture.

WHAT IS OPTIMUM POSTURE?

Optimum posture is when the body is mechanically aligned with minimum strain on the muscles, ligaments, and joints. In this efficient position the fewest restrictions are imposed on the muscular and nervous systems, energy is not wasted to simply hold the body up.

This energy can be utilized for creativity and productivity. Optimum posture consists of a combination of the following: chin lock, neutral spine, core engagement, sternum lift, shoulder blade retraction, joint mobility, muscle flexibility, and diaphragmatic breathing.

BENEFITS OF OPTIMUM POSTURE:

• Decreased stress and tension in the supportive skeletal muscles

• Less wear and tear in the joint structures

• Increased contracting/relaxing ability of the diaphragm enhancing the amount of air capacity in the lungs

• More flexibility in joint movement

• Reduced strain on the neck, jaw, and upper back muscles

• Increased amount of energy

• More positive, confident self-image

• Relaxed state of mind, carrying the body effortlessly

Basic Rules about Stretching

NO BOUNCING: Hold a static stretch to build up soft tissue tension so change occurs in tissue length. Bouncing can tear tissues or cause injuries in other affected areas.

NO PAIN: Stretching should not cause a sensation of discomfort; sharp pain, particularly, indicates that the muscle is being stretched too far.

DO NOT HOLD THE BREATH: Relax, breathe slowly and rhythmically, and focus on the muscles when stretching. Lengthen and stretch the muscle tissue upon exhalation.

KNOW WHAT AREA NEEDS TO BE STRETCHED AND WHY: Each individual requires different areas of flexibility. Assessments are helpful to recognize the tight, unstable areas, and appropriate stretches need to be prescribed. Maintain a balance between stretching and strengthening exercises to insure joint stability, minimizing the chance of joint injury.

WATCH FOR MUSCLE SUBSTITUTION: Be specific on the muscle group being stretched. Make sure that compensatory muscle groups are not overpowering.

GENERAL STRETCHING TIPS : Stretching the muscle groups is only beneficial when done correctly. Just as there is more than one way to achieve a set goal, there is more than one stretch to enhance flexibility.

Based upon our experiences, gradual, slow, sustained stretches, reaching away, using correct technique prevents injuries from occurring. Stretch to the point of moderate tension and maintain the stretch for a minimum of 30 – 45 seconds, preferably 45 seconds – 1 ½ minutes.

Relax for 5 – 10 seconds between stretches and repeat on the other side. Spend additional time stretching muscles that are chronically tight.

Perform 2 – 3 sets per stretch, time permitting, repeating the stretch on the same muscle group. Once the body is warmed up, stretches may be held for longer periods of time.

Asana Hatha yoga benfits

Yoga is a different physical workout than normal exercise; It is also related to the relation of meditation and inner conscience. It is defined as the holding of a pose or maintaining the body in a position for a period. Asanas are very useful for maintaining good health.

Type of Asanas:

Stretching posture: It should be done with care.They cleanse the nerves and provide relief from chronic diseases.

Pranayama Asana: This is done while breathing and exhaling,hence, these are known as Pranayama asanas, and this asana purifies the blood.

Asana, which requires force: in this type, some weight is lifted or force is required; This increases strength.

Asanas, which activate nerves: There are selective asanas, which are performed rapidly and repeatedly, which help to activate nerves, and also purify the body.

Depending on how the posture is performed,they are classified as follows:

Asana while standing

Sitting Asana

Reverse Asanas

Asanas as soon as they lie on the ground

Benefits of yoga:

This helps to keep the spine flexible.

It helps the body to cleanse the glands and remove harmful foreign particles from the body.

By doing the asana the blood vessels do not harden and the heart remains strong.

It helps to strengthen muscles and improve body composition.

It helps in the awakening of the Kundalini in the spinal column and refreshes the mind, and one becomes energetic.

It strengthens the digestive system by cleaning the intestines,stomach and other parts of the body.

Asana provides good health to both mind and body.

Key points while doing the Asanas:

It should be done in a quiet and peaceful place with proper hygiene.For meditation, the person may feel good by using the fragrance.

This should be done on a plain ground where a blanket or dari extends.

This should be done for a minimum of 15 minutes and a maximum of 30 minutes.

It should be left once a week; One can go swimming or walking instead of the posture.

The best time for posture is in the morning, but it can also be done in the evening.

Yoga asana should be done on an empty stomach, it can be done 4 to 5 hours after a meal or 2 hours after a light meal.

The asana should begin with prayer or meditation and end with Shavasana.

There should not be strong wind on the body while doing the asana.

One should cross-check while performing an asana properly. And asana should be done in proper order.

After doing the asana, one should rest for half an hour and then take a glass of milk and fruits.

There is a physical foundation from hatha yoga in all yoga activities.This forms the basis for all other yoga and science.The many paths of yoga that have been carried out,combine foundational principles from Hatha Yoga. It is designed to purify and strengthen the body. Many yogis first become integral to hatha yoga, then as their body specializes in discipline,they move towards a more challenging and demanding style of yoga. They do this to awaken the mind and soul completely.

According to Hatha Yoga in Sanskrit, "ha" means sun while "tha" means moon. Also, the word "yoga" is meant to be a union or power.Hatha yoga is considered to be the more scientific path of yoga and includes a basic triad. This is to encourage complete transformation of the body, as well as the mind; Furthermore, the words used for asana / mudra are asana, breath control or pranayama; Then finally the technique of clearance or refinement.

Most yoga instructors and practitioners in other parts of the world can choose to modify Hatha yoga asanas to suit their different fitment levels.This method of modifying Hatha Yoga, is not accepted by other yoga style purists. Asanas can be very simple. This can be as easy as lying on the floor,or it may involve twisting, as well as pulling.Once a student becomes accustomed to physical discipline, a new height of awareness will be attained through concentration and meditation.Hatha yoga can be traced to a great extent, so that a restless mind can be controlled properly, stress can be reduced and enjoyment of peace can also be possible. Here are the eight paths

1. Yama: Pursuit of truth, ethics as well as personal conduct

2. Niyama: Fall of ego, satisfaction

3. Asana Fixed posture

4. Pranayama– Proper Breathing exercises for control of prana

5. Pratyahara: withdrawl of human senses

6. Dhyan: meditation

7. Dharna: Perfection

8. Samadhi: Experiencing the divine

Benefits of Hatha Yoga

Hatha yoga can provide many benefits.This can have emotional, physical as well as mental benefits.

Physical improvements can be highlighted as

• help improves digestion

• strengthen the muscles

• Provides spine and joints flexibility

• Increase oxygen flow along with blood flow

• Offer better body balance and posture

As stated earlier, practicing Hatha Yoga also has an emotional impact on proper practice. Although they may differ, those who have practiced and are dedicated to discipline have made claims to experience:

• Stress Relief

• deep relaxation and good sleep

• Increased ability to concentrate completely

• consciousness and awareness

Precaution doing Asanas:

If someone is suffering from colitis, one should not do asana, in which the spine is bent.

If someone's eyes are red, he should not head.

An asana should be stopped at the point when it is tired.

Women should not perform Siddhasana or Mayurasan.

If someone is suffering from heart diseases, he should do asana only after consulting a doctor.

Benefits of Surya Namaskar

10 minutes of Surya Namaskar daily is highly beneficial for body and mind, here's how If you find yourself as a part of the same equation, well, fret not! You barely need to take out multiple hours to stay fit. All you need is to look beyond earth to solve your problem. Towards the sun, perhaps?

Sun Salutation: How Surya Namaskar can change various aspects of your life?

Sun has been a source of both spirituality and vitality on the Earth since time immemorial. Its significance can be traced from Mayan, Egyptian, Aztec, Tibetan, and Indian civilizations to the ones that emerged later. Spirituality apart, there is also a logical reason behind the sun's prominence.

Scientifically, the sun radiates energy to the earth in the form of heat and sunlight – without which life couldn't have sustained here. Sparing just 10 minutes for yourself every day can have dramatic changes in various aspects of your life. Hence, Surya Namaskar, or Sun Salutation, has a range of effects on the human body.

Primarily, it ingrains discipline within you. Although you might be having an erratic schedule – shifting from board meetings to late-night assignments, brainstorming sessions to business development initiatives, and so on – devoting time to Surya Namaskar every morning ensures that you have a set schedule which cannot be altered. It brings greater stability to your life despite the sheer dynamism prevailing in it.

Secondly, it is a full-body workout. Guess how many calories do you burn after a mix of 30-minute exercises? Weightlifting burns around 199 calories, tennis around 232 calories, football around 298 calories, rock climbing around 364 calories, and running around 414 calories.

Now, guess how much calories does Surya Namaskar burn?

So, technically, 10 minutes of Surya Namaskar translates into burning 139 calories, which is more than what you'd burn even after swimming for 10 minutes. Surya Namaskar, also known as 'The Ultimate Asana', strengthens your back as well as your muscles and brings down blood sugar levels. It also improves metabolism and blood circulation (hence, a glowing skin) and ensures regular menstrual cycle for women.

Surya Namaskar consists of 7 asanas that are performed in a cyclic order, thereby creating 12 asanas in total. They are as follows:

Pranamasana: Surya Namaskar begins by greeting the Sun God in a prayer position while standing upright. It helps in calming down your body and mind.

Hastauttanasana: In this asana, hands are gradually lifted and the back is bent backwards. Slowly inhale air and bring your biceps close to the ears. The asana helps in stretching your chest as well as abdomen and surges the energy flow towards the upper part of your body.

Padahastasana: After stretching your abdominal region, Padahastasana further massages your belly. Doing so improves digestion while also enhancing your blood flow to the brain. Just exhale, bend, and try touching the floor with your hands while keeping your spine straight. Make sure that you exhale slowly and thoroughly. The asana also plays a role in eliminating female disorders.

Ashwa Sanchalanasana: This asana stretches your spine further along with quadriceps and iliopsoas muscles. It also stimulates your abdominal organs. After Padahastasana, start bending your knees towards the right side of your chest while moving your left leg backwards. You can take support from the ground. Raise your head and look forward. Also, inhale throughout.

Parvatasana: It makes your arms and legs stronger and relieves varicose veins. Parvatasana also stretches calf and spine muscles. Breathe out and lift your waist to make an 'inverted V' with your body. Try to keep your heels on the ground.

Dandasana: The dandasana improves body posture and reinforces your back muscles and spine. It also stretches your shoulder and chest. You have to take your parvatasana pose forward and perform a plank while inhaling. Make sure that both of your hands are just below your shoulders and the body is parallel to the ground.

Ashtanga Namaskara: Ashtanga Namaskara asana also helps in strengthening your chest, arms, and legs. Exhale and bring your chin down on the ground. Keep your hips up in the air. Your chin, chest, hands, and knees must be on the ground.

Bhujangasana: Now, slowly bring your hip down and place your legs as well as midsection on the ground while inhaling. Keep your head up and bend your back. Your body posture will resemble a cobra in this asana.   It   relieves   tension   from   the   back   and   spine.

Parvatasana: Keeping up with the cyclic order, repeat parvatasana.

Ashwa Sanchalanasana: Repeat Ashwa Sanchalanasana by lunging with your left leg forward this time.

Padahastasana: Repeat Padahastasana.

Hastauttanasana: Repeat Hastauttanasana.

The ideal time to perform Surya Namaskar is during sunrise while facing towards the sun.

Remember, Surya Namaskar can be performed with your day-to-day food intake. However, it is always good to embrace a Sattvik diet. If Satvik diet is a bit too much for you, you can also look towards a Rajasik diet while avoiding Tamsik food and beverages.

Lastly, Surya Namaskar is known to have several psychological benefits as well. The physical exercise has a visible impact on memory retention, anxiety, and even helps in battling insomnia.

Just imagine, all of this happens by merely devoting 10 minutes of your day to Surya Namaskar. After all, the sun is the source and bearer of life on earth. We must all seek good health from the sun.

Benefits of doing Yoga in the Morning

Everyone knows how much it is beneficial to do yoga in the morning and it is also able to keep you away from many types of diseases. It always keeps you fresh and healthy.There are ways to do yoga, although you can practice yoga anytime and at any time. But doing yoga in the morning is considered more effective. Today you are studying Yoga for Health.

Now a days lot of people are doing yoga in the morning.And while there's no doubt that regular flows come with their fair share of benefits—better sleep, more flexibility, reduced anxiety—the time at which you're doing yoga is also very fruitful.

Whether you're a sunrise sweat warrior or prefer a post-work savasana, there are different feel-good properties associated with doing yoga in the morning and at night. Because of that, you may want to switch up your style depending on your schedule.

Yoga in the morning

Waking up and flowing through some sun salutations is a great way to set the tone for the day ahead. Studies have shown its effectiveness for reducing anxiety, and a few easy poses in the early morning can help you get into a positive frame of mind for the day ahead.

Yoga keeps you calm in every way and increases the energy in the body as well as helps in keeping you relaxed. It connects you to yourself.In this article, we are telling you today what kind of benefits you get from doing yoga in the morning and how it is considered the most effective time to do yoga. Read the benefits of Yoga in the Morning in this article.

Keep the process of sleep and hormones right

If you practice yoga in the morning every day, then it keeps your sleep process right.

It exerts good effect on our endocrine system in the body.

Because of which it also keeps the hormone easily by balancing.

It regulates the melatonin, a hormone that induces sleep in the body.

Keeps healthy

It has been proved in a study that people who get up early in the morning and exercise, they are more healthy.

These people also do not get tired more than other people and they feel fresh all day.

It is advisable to do yoga postures before 6 am.

Increases metabolism

Metabolism increases in the body by doing yoga in the morning daily.

It also keeps your digestive system healthy.

Fat decreases quickly due to increase in metabolism in the body.

If you do yoga in the morning, then the fat of the stomach also decreases very quickly.

Also, by doing yoga in the morning, your body gets energy for the whole day.

Works like caffeine

By doing yoga in the morning, it acts like caffeine in the body.

The flow of oxygen in the body and circulation of blood in the body is smooth.

Wakes your brain and makes you feel fresh.

As you wake up in the morning and drink tea or coffee and feel free, make yoga your morning habit.

Doing yoga in the morning makes us more energetic and increase our productivity.

Keeps away from laziness

When you do yoga in the morning, it gives good stretching to your body.

Due to this stretching, you can keep yourself away from laziness throughout the day.

Also you are able to do your tasks quickly.

With the practice of yoga, you make your body flexible and muscles of your body become quite strong.

Your body is able to remain active throughout the day due to this.In this article above, we told you today that if you practice yoga in the morning, it will prove to be beneficial for you.

Morning Routine for healthy Skin

After sleep has refreshed and healed your body, the morning hours can do wonders for your skin, if planned well.

Drink water

Start your day by drinking one glass of water. Nothing can work better than hydrating your skin right in the morning.

Breakfast

Never skip breakfast. In fact, your breakfast should be rich in nutrients and should include fruits, oats, multi-grain breads and dry fruits for a healthy body and skin.

Drink green tea or detox water to flush the body toxins away before taking a bath.

Yoga

Yoga is beneficial for the skin and the body. A 5-minute face yoga session will improve circulation, facilitating the delivery of oxygen and nutrients and relieve tension in the facial muscles.

Sarvangasana, chakrasana, dhanurasana, shirshasana are effective in increasing blood flow to the skin and removing toxins.Pranayam stimulates endocrine gland, oxygenate cells reducing stress, and improving blood flow for skin glow. Practice kapalbhati, bhastrika, and anulom-vilom.

Skincare rituals

Your morning skincare routine should include cleansing, moisturizing and protection. Use a cleanser that is rich in aloe vera and other skin-nourishing ingredients. Don't forget to apply sunscreen when you step out.

Splash fresh rose water on face and eyes stored in a silver vessel.

In the morning, remove toxins accumulated in the body during sleep, oil pulling will detoxify, keep the facial skin healthy and is a good exercise for the mouth, jawline, and maintains perfect dental health.

Tongue cleaning to remove accumulated phlegm, according to ancient texts, helps you receive nutrients smoothly.

Remove your makeup before taking a bath. This will prevent the harsh rubbing of skin that can irritate the area around the eyes. This also ensures deeper cleansing of the ski'.

Home remedies

Apply a 'mukh lepam' before bathing for 10 minutes while you are doing your daily chores. Black lentil powdered and blended with warm milk or clarified butter is an idle morning team. On weekends highly recommended is a body scrub. Keep a body scrub powder made of orange peels, green gram, rice powder in a jar and mix it with milk and coconut oil, let it dry and scrub in the opposite direction and finally wash off.

On weekdays, preserve the skin's moisture by dabbing shower oil on wet cleansed skin, natural cold-pressed oils in shower oil are very nourishing, softening and seal the natural moisture.

Use face masks for glowing skin. You can use a turmeric, besan or gram flour face pack for brighter and clearer skin. You can also use a tomato or potato peel to get rid of red and tanned skin.

Facial exercises

Thirty minutes before a shower, d' facial exercises. 'Kiss the ceiling' is the best way to tone almost all facial muscles, 'pinching' the jawline and neck is another very beneficial exercise to remove stiffness, improve blood flow to the skin.

Self-massage before bath also moisturizes the skin and gives a beautiful sheen.

Wellness Bring a warm natural glow to the skin by removing negative emotions, toxins from your mind.

Breathing Basics Revive

Feel the calmness the smoothness within the body while breathing.This process of controlled and proper breathing we term it as the reawakening of the inner self with which we link the energy flow of the divine.

Here I am talking of one way of breathing

To begin with sit in an ideal place you are comfortable with.The place should be clean ,proper ventilation,good quality of oxygen should flow.Morning period on sunrise is the best time to breathe.If it is not possible follow the process at evening time.Calm your mind.Let no disturbance occurs internally or externally.

When the things has settled now start breathing.The process should be slow,very slow.The sound of breath shouldn't be heard even by our ears infact only be felt by us.

Stop the breath when it is full taken between the eyes or at the forhead.For the first phase Breath stop time should be equal to the time taken for taking breath inwards.

Now exhale the breath with the same time as the inhalation process.Stop for the same time.

Repeat the process but REMEMBER the stopping time should increase every time on or after breathing.i.e breathe in – stop – breathe out – stop.Stopping time should increase from as example from 10 to 20 to 30 seconds and say on as long as you continue.

If in initial stages if it is not possibleto go beyond 30 or 40 seconds(stopping breath)repeat the process of breathing to the same period of the last breath stop taken.

Do this process of breathing for 25 to 30 minutes daily.

Yes within few weeks you will realise the wonderful effects.

Not only headache but the divine power of healing in the body has started.The tiny roots of healing is there.It will show you its effect making to believe in a more positive balanced ways.The fear of unknown will disappear,legitimacy of existence will flower.

Proper breathing is a natural healing process.Remember here divinity is in the process of stoppage and the flow of breathing.

Stoppage has an end to flow and the flow has an end to stoppage of the breath.

Repetitive process of breathing is a joy.An amazing experience of hope and journey ahead, a solution of idelogical conflicts we face,awakening of our soul we are bound to be blessed with.

How to do Anulom Vilom Pranayam

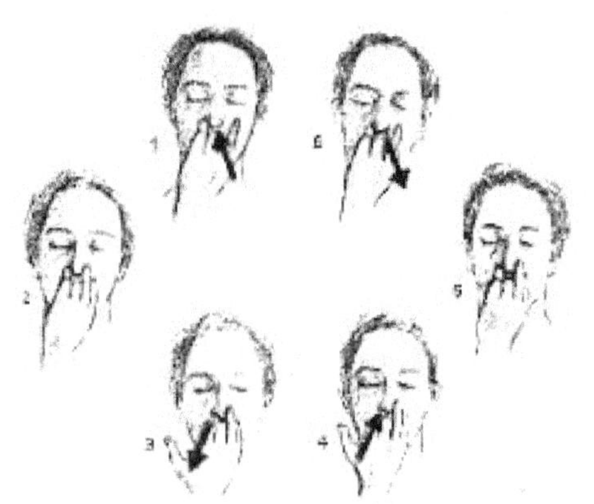

Anulom Vilom pranayama is really very helpful for our health. It is very effective for body purification. Anulom Vilom is an excellent breathing technique to calm and center the mind while improving blood circulation.

Anulom vilom pranayam, also called the alternate nostril breathing technique, is an incredible energiser, which works effectively to relieve stress and anxiety.

Regular practitioners have also treated their serious health conditions that include heart problems, cartilage, depression, asthma, high blood pressure and arthritis.

Yoga Expert suggests practising anulom vilom to be the best breathing exercise to manage stress levels as it helps one take control of breathing and thereby, control the mind.

To do the Anulom Vilom Pranayam, sit cross-legged with the neck and spine straight.Ensure that you are comfortable. The right hand should be in gyan mudra (join the tip of the thumb and index finger) and the left hand should be in pranayam mudra (close the index and middle finger).

 Close your eyes and the right nostril with the thumb of the right hand and inhale through the left and exhale through right, inhale through right and exhale through left. Repeat a few times and relax.

Deep Relaxation may also have health Benefits

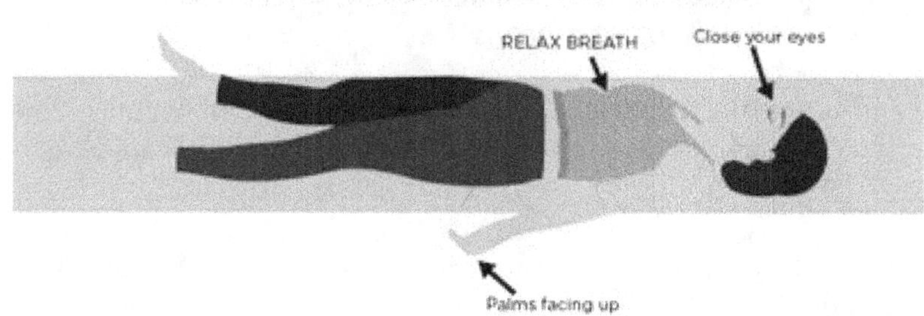

Many yoga sessions end with Corpse Pose (Savasana), which is a pose meant to create deep relaxation. This pose is very important for integrating the benefits of the breath and movement practices, and should not be skipped. Plus, if you're feeling ungrounded, deep relaxation may help your nervous system rebalance itself.

It has also observed that sometimes people who have mental health issues aren't always comfortable doing deep relaxation for too long, or they start feeling fidgety. But even if you only practice Corpse Pose for a minute or two, you will reap some of its calming benefits. In the traditional Corpse Pose, you lie flat on your back with your legs resting hip distance apart and your arms relaxed alongside your body with your palms facing up.

One relaxation exercise you can do in Corpse Pose is to focus on one part of your body at a time. While lying on your back, bring your awareness to your left foot, then your left shin, then your left knee, until you have covered every major part of your body. When you finish this deep relaxation, consider doing a very short meditation.You can do this while still lying in Corpse Pose, or sitting up.I suggests doing a "my favorite place" meditation, where you pick an image that brings you joy and mentally take yourself there. See the sights, smell the smells, feel the sensations. For people with mental health issues, this type of meditation is preferable to letting a teacher mentally guide you to places like a beach or a mountain, because certain images such as a beach or a mountain may be triggering.

Find a Yoga Teacher With Mental Health Expertise

You can practice yoga on your own, but having a teacher who has experience instructing people with mental health issues is especially valuable for someone with schizophrenia. These teachers are likely to be certified in yoga therapy, as opposed to being a more basic yoga teacher.

If you can afford a few private sessions, this might be better than diving into a group class.If you are feeling anxious, for example, your teacher can modify the practice so you don't do as much movement that day, or, if you're not feeling grounded, the teacher might have you spend a lot of time sitting on the floor with both pelvic bones touching the ground.

Pran Yoga will infuse Life energy in You

The power of life is known as "Prana". The word creature was coined due to the existence of life in living beings. The higher the amount of life element in a creature, the more powerful, advanced and great it becomes.

At the same time, the higher the amount of life in which a creature becomes weak, the useless, lazy and low level. The main feeling of life inside the body is considered to be its 'Tejasvita'. Its meaning is found in the Gayatri Mantra with the word 'bharga'. The word bharga means 'fast'.

In order to increase the level of life in humans, it is considered best to practice 'Pranayama'. Diet, systematic routine, relaxed and calm mind, happy mind and celibacy all these work to increase the power of life in you.

The increase of vital energy in the body means to fill that wonderful element inside itself through which the powers of human beings develop further. Through this, age can also be increased. Come, let's read Prana Yoga in today's article.

The effect of Pran Yoga does not remain confined to our body only, but its effect makes all the senses and the senses powerful in us, by eliminating the negativity inside the mind and awakening the feeling of positiveness and creativity in it. In addition, it also gives the seeker a feeling of happiness, happiness and joy. With this, the intellect of the person develops rapidly and the body always remains healthy.

Here are the few ways to gain prana within you

Kumbhak kriya

It involves breathing in a controlled motion.Whenever breathing is done slowly and rapidly while doing pranayama, it is necessary to have a rhythm and proportion.Holding the breath drawn inside is called Kumbhak.

The action of stopping the breath in the body is called internal Kumbhak.When the breath is exhaled, it is called external Kumbhak.

In this action also it is necessary to have rhythm and proportion.

Rechak kriya

The action of exhaling the breath taken in a controlled motion is called Rechak kriya.When breathing exits in any manner, it is necessary to have rhythm and proportion.

Omkar

The word is actually considered to be Brahma i.e. God. By doing this, all diseases are destroyed.With its regular practice, the mind becomes calm and pure, as well as all mental disorders and bad thoughts run away from it.To perform this pranayama, the word Om is chanted while closing your eyes and taking a deep breath.

Anulom Vilom

To do Anulom Vilom pranayama, one of the nostrils is closed with fingers and the breath is filled through the second nostril.The same action is then repeated from the second orifice of the nose in the same way.Not only does this pranayama clean the nose, it also brings peace to the restless mind and it proves quite beneficial in relieving mental troubles.

Kapalbhati Pranayam

This Kapalbhati Pranayama is formed by the combination of the words Kapala and Bhati. The meaning of the skull is the head and the meaning of the sister is shining.While doing this pranayama, you sit up straight and fast release your breath in such a way that your stomach feels inward.But keep in mind that during this time your focus should not be on your stomach, but instead of going in and out of your breath.

By doing Kapalabhati Pranayam, the digestive system is strengthened and lungs are also strong, as well as it is very beneficial in diabetes and ophthalmology.

Ujjayi Pranayam

Ujjayi literally means sea and during this pranayama, the sea-like sound is extracted from the breath and this is why this pranayama is named as Ujjayi Pranayam.While doing this pranayama, the breath is stopped in the neck and during this time the sound of the sea is taken out.

Shambhavi Pranayam

It is believed that by doing this pranayama, the third eye can be awakened.In this posture, the space between the two eyebrows, called the command cycle, is developed.By doing this, the mind becomes sharp, the eyes glow and the confidence also increases.

To do this pranayama, sit down with the neck and back straight and keep the hands on your knees, concentrate your attention on your obedience in this posture.

Sheetali Pranayam

Sheetali Pranayama is named after the word Sheetal. Cold means cold.By doing Sheetali Pranayama, the mind of the seeker calms down as well as excessive heat present in the body is also removed.Blood pressure is also controlled by performing this pranayama.If you are in a state of tension, you can relieve your stress by doing Sheetali Pranayam for just 10 minutes.

To perform this pranayama,you twists your tongue and inhales and is released.

Nadishodhan Pranayam

By regular practice of pulse purification pranayama, the blood of your body clears and the amount of oxygen inside the blood also increases.By doing this pranayama, all the dirt is removed from the veins of the body, hence this pranayama is called Nadihodhan Pranayam.

This pranayama makes your entire respiratory system strong and at the same time doing it relieves problems like restlessness and headache.

With meditation find freedom from attachment

In the practical life the things that are useful or purposeful for us, only the inner conscious can find the answer to it. Eating, drinking and living in peace are all for the fulfillment of our mental well being.

Important thing is that the reasoning or logical thinking is related to our Consciousness. So it is to be justified that spiritualism can be attained relating to human's Conscious level of his sense of mindfulness.

By regular practice of Sadhna or meditation a human being can find his true path of spiritual enlightenment. The pure state of bliss is one such philosophy.

By following spiritual practices we will find the true state of blissness or pure happiness that is permanent and absolute and cannot be find with any other means, but only with the way of following spiritual practices.

According to our Conscious level we can find real knowledge of destruction or development. With the increase in level of our Consciousness we start to find happiness, beginning from small segment or section to holistic level of inner joy that we call as the state of blissness.

In this process we start to find happiness and give preference to deep mental peace rather than any physical pleasure of desires and attachments. We tend to leave these pleasures aside.

Attachments and desires causes attraction that diverts our attention and act as hindrance towards our spiritual growth. These desires gives birth to a new desire on completion of previous desires.

For Country's love or any such rare happiness a human do not fear to surrender or give his life for it. There are thousands of such examples in history. This is human's higher level of Consciousness or a healthy mindset.

By the practice of Ashtanga Yoga a devotee or practitioner can slowly and steadily grow his thinking power and with that developed thinking he can find spiritual awakening. By this spiritual awakening he can find true happiness.

We should know that without natural knowledge it is not possible to do so. We should increase to raise allegiance or fidelity. By inclination only, allegiance will rise and with growth of the allegiance we will be blessed by god's Grace.

With only a little of God's Grace we find freedom from attachment with this physical structure or body. Perpetual perversion discretion is awakened and this discretion develops us to Brahmroop or immortal. It is to be noted that In meditation route, the biggest thing is devotion or allegiance.

How to begin the practice of meditation

Sit down with leg crossed, back straight and eyes closed. Beware of your breath around the nostrils, as you breathe in and as you breathe out. Breathe in, experiencing the whole body, breathe out, experiencing the whole body. Breathe in, relaxing the whole body, breathe out, relaxing the whole body..Always mindful, breathe in, mindful, breathe out. Open your eyes and come out of meditation.

How to begin your practice ?

Begin with a short period of 10-15 minutes. Slowly increase the duration. One hour is a good span for daily meditatin.

Benefits

• Sooths and calms the mind

• Relieves tension and anxiety

• Helps to reduce high blood pressure

• Effective for insomnia

• Improves concentration

• Builds self-confidence

Keeping in line with meditation can greatly increase the effectiveness of the process, as you can not only learn to perform better but also strengthen your mind's ability to concentrate and calm down.

When you can experience the positive benefits of meditation, repeated practice not only helps keep your mind calm for longer, but also enables you to gain a greater degree of mental clarity and well being.

Warm up and Cool Down

WARM UP : Warming up the body by increasing the blood circulation and heart rate is an essential part of yoga. Although some individuals use the Sun Salutation as a warm-up in yoga, if convenient, we recommend a 10 – 12 minute warm-up consisting of a brisk walk, cycling, running, etc. The warm-up should be intense enough to increase body temperature, to warm up the muscles and cause a slight sweat but not cause any fatigue.

THE BENEFITS OF WARMING UP

• Increase body and tissue temperature.

• Increase blood flow through the active muscles

• Increase the heart rate, preparing the cardiovascular system for work

• Increase the exchange rate of oxygen and carbon dioxide from hemoglobin in the blood

• Increase the speed at which nerve impulses travel, facilitating body movements

• Increase reciprocal innervation efficiency, allowing muscles to contract and relax faster and more efficiently

• Decrease muscular tension

• Enhance the ability of connective tissue to elongate

COOL DOWN : The cool-down period is just as important as the warm up. The cool-down period helps the body return to its pre-yoga practice state, a small investment of time for the many benefits received.A minimum quiet down of half hour is usually recommended when every yoga session.

THE BENEFITS OF COOL DOWN

• Help clear the muscles of accumulated lactic acid

• Lessen excessive fatigue

• Reduce soreness and cramps

• Keep muscles from tightening up

• Lower blood pressure

• come the temperature back to resting levels

• Restore the center rate to a resting level in brief, a relax speeds overall recovery in preparation for succeeding yoga sessions. A cool down is also helpful to relax and unwind the mind, a transition from the intensity of the yoga session to the day-to-day activities. Cooling down is a wonderful way to re-align or re-position the body's postural mechanics.Maintaining this posture for at least 10 – 15 minutes re-educates the body (hardware) and mind (software) to adapt to this comfortable, stress-free posture.

Yoga & meditation for Spiritual Enlightenment

All of us can sense the greatness we have within.In Buddhism it is called the Buddha Nature, and within Christianity, Christ Consciousness. Call it what you will, it is there and requires no perfecting on our part to make it perfect.

The trouble is we not only don't see it, but we believe that meditation, yoga, and other spiritual exercises produce it. We think such things as, "I will meditate to awaken my mind," as if the pure fundamental consciousness within needs awakening.

We may do so with the best intentions, yet not realize that joining a meditation class or yoga studio may be counterproductive to achieving our spiritual ambitions. Working to become more aware and in tune with the nature of reality works under the assumptions that we are not in tune and that a certain amount of perfecting is necessary to become enlightened—or at least achieve a far greater awareness than we presently know.

As soon as we meditate or practice a yoga sequence, it is natural that a performer of these actions emerges, just as it does in everything in life.

If we study in college and receive a degree, we have accomplished something, and we cannot escape the fact that we are enjoying the results of our effort. We cannot close a business deal and escape the sense of accomplishing something.

In everything we do, there is a doer. This model works well within the conventions of the ordinary affairs of life, but we get into trouble when the attitude of "doer" gets into our spiritual enterprise.

One of the biggest obstacles to the realization of the aims of meditation and yoga is meditation and yoga, which may seem ridiculous, but is nevertheless true. It is not the aim of spiritual discipline to achieve something, but rather to see something within that we have not properly noticed before.

When we strive to achieve something, we immediately start covering over the very thing we wish to see because we start concocting an image of what it is supposed to be. We may visualize different colored lights shining forth from our chakras, or a blazing white light between our brows, or a shining Buddha or Christ in our heart, all of which may emerge, but they certainly won't as long as we are trying to make them do so.

If it were true that meditation and yoga cover over and obscure their aim, why bother with a meditation and yoga practice? The simple answer is because there is nothing better.

Since so few of us can sit down and allow perfect awareness to arise, we have techniques to help us do so. But, these techniques have to be properly used, which is often not the case. Why not? Because capable and realized instructors are rare, and few take the time to thoroughly study authentic texts that lay forth in clear terms the merely expedient nature of spiritual techniques, yoga and meditation, and so forth.

If there were any aim to spiritual disciplines, it would be to help us stop getting in our way and allow what is already perfect within to shine. Allowing is what is meant by the "effortless path," a term often used in Vajrayana Buddhism. But effortlessness actually requires a lot of effort; it is not easy to break the habit of "doer" and sit back and allow realization to arise.

We must make ourselves vulnerable to realization, and part of being vulnerable is getting rid of the notion of achiever. We don't achieve anything when we attain illumination but only recognize, finally, what has been there all along.

A story is told in Buddhism to help those struggling toward realization to understand "effortlessness." Suppose a loving parent sending her child off into the world wishes to safeguard that child from misfortune.

She lovingly sews within his coat a valuable jewel and sends him off. The child knows nothing of the jewel and wanders throughout the world, enduring much hardship. Years pass, and one day he finally discovers the jewel, which makes all his ambitions possible.

In a Buddhist sutra, the Avatamsaka Sutra, it is said: "All living beings have the Buddha Nature, but false thinking and attachments obscure it." In other words, the jewel—our Buddha Nature—is there always shining, but we don't see it because we are too busy trying to.

We are attached to the thought that we can achieve enlightenment as if it were a produced state of mind, rather than an innate one, and exert a good deal of effort trying to achieve it. All of this is an activity, and all activity is counterproductive, whether it is physical or mental. What we need to learn is how to be still.

Strangely, being still—body and mind—is elusive. Being inactive is more difficult than any activity. Not applying effort is more challenging than applying it.

Proper meditation seldom involves doing anything other than what we are doing. Are we trying to accomplish something, or are we trying to get out of our own way? A small shift in attitude can make all the difference in the world. If we can shift our view from achieving enlightenment to recognizing enlightenment, we make ourselves vulnerable to awakening and grace.

Some may remember the autosterograms that were popular about 20 years ago—those art books full of pages that at first glance appeared as just a confusion of dots, but an image would emerge if you looked at the page without trying to see anything.

Not surprisingly, kids were far better than adults because of their innocent minds. In a similar manner, if we can meditate free of ideas of what is or is not, realization of what has been there all along will emerge.

Awareness during Asana Practice

There are 4 sequential ways to direct awareness during asana practice:

BODY : The awareness is focused on the actual physical movements, the interaction between the various components of the body, i.e. bones, joints, ligaments, muscles, abdominal organs, etc. This method of practice includes single-pointedness in the physical body.

MIND : The focus is placed on disassociating from the thoughts arising in the mind as the body stretches further into the asana.

BREATH : The body and mind focuses are integrated through breath. In addition to the awareness of physical and mental movements described above, individual movements are synchronized with the breath. The movements become slower, which in turn slows the brain waves, increasing the breath capacity, further enhancing relaxation and awareness.

SOUND : The final practice is to coordinate and integrate the following: reaching with the body, stilling the mind, enhancing the breath, and releasing sound. In each asana in Sound Body YOGA the breath is exhaled on the mantra 'AUM', uniting all the participants with one sound and synchronous breath.

Tuladandasana –balancing stick Pose

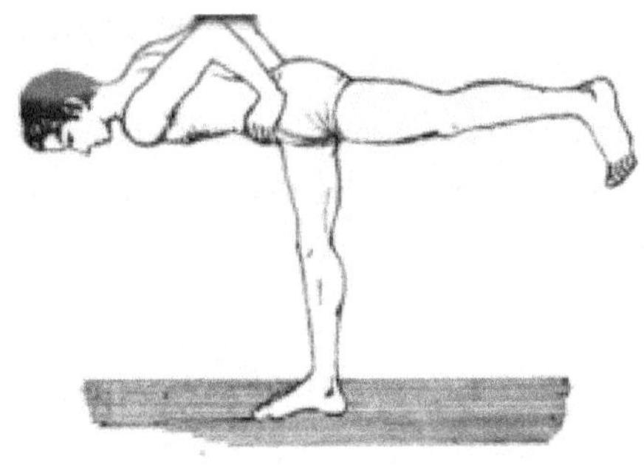

Tuladandasana is a complicated reconciliation position which needs stability, focus and core strength. The name comes from the Sanskritic language tula, that means "balance"; danda, that means "stick" or "staff"; and position, that means "pose."

In this position, the body forms a "T." The arms square measure raised overhead with the palms facing one another or touching. the rear leg lifts off the bottom, the anchored leg is straight, and also the arms, body part and back leg square measure parallel with the bottom.

Tuladandasana is also ordinarily named in English as reconciliation stick create. The position is additionally generally referred to as Virabhadrasana three (warrior 3 or flying person pose) or eka padasana (one-legged pose).

If there was ever a cause to focus in the mind of a runner, Tuladandasana (or equalization stick pose) is it. With four ten-second bursts of pulse-racing intensity, the cause usually seems like ninety per cent mind : ten per cent matter.

Like most yoga postures, this cause needs a powerful core and a unprecedented quantity of focus. whether or not it's throughout a lung-busting 5K or a marathon, we've all had introspection, 'why am I doing this?' moments once running feels like a extremely silly plan.Tuladandasana is like sprinting the last 400m of a 5K race – you've to dig deep, keep calm and breathe.

Tuladandasana: Step by Step

1. Stand along with your feet along, heels and toes touching, arms by your facet.

2. Interlace your fingers, emotional the index fingers (so you are virtually doing a 'gun' hand gesture , and keeping your arms fast, raise them on top of your head therefore your striated muscle are tucked behind your ears. Relax your shoulders to avoid them hunching.

3. Take a leap forward along with your right foot, keeping your toe pointed and your quad narrowed to drag up the knee cap.

4. Inhale, tighten your abdomen muscles and your glutes and slowly tip forward, eupneic as your left leg comes off the ground and extends out behind you. Keep rotating forward till you are equalization sort of a majuscule 'T', along with your arms before of you and left leg out behind you, each narrowed.

5. to assist your balance and open your chest, keep your gaze forward and avoid tucking your chin to your chest. Keep your hips level by slightly rotating your left hip in and down therefore it's level along with your right hip. Your right leg ought to be fast the total time.

6. As it's 'only' a 10 second posture (repeated doubly on every leg), it's tempting to carry your breath, however doing therefore can cause you to feel dizzy and probably even unwholesome, therefore keep your respiratory steady and controlled.

Exit the posture constant means you went in, and come back to standing posture before continuation on the left leg.

Tuladandasana: the advantages

'This posture sounds very easy, 'but do not be fooled. The forward tilt of your body part sends high-speed blood speeding towards the center, that elevates your pulse. it is not the least bit uncommon to feel terribly out of breath when this cause.'

'The second set will be extremely difficult, and staying calm and respiratory steady is that the solely thanks to get through it. In running terms, it's like doing speedwork: If you target however exhausting the ultimate set are and the way a lot of your calves can burn subsequently, you will not be setting up a hundred per cent.

keep calm and conceive to the posture (remember it's solely ten seconds) and you may develop a strength of mind that you simply will then use to enhance your running.'

Health benefit of Sarvang Asana

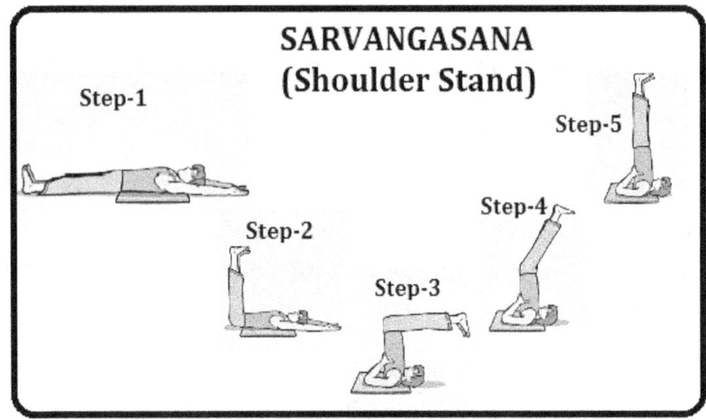

BENEFITS

• Stretches the entire spine

• Improves circulation of blood in the lower extremity

• Massages abdominal organs

• Stimulates the glandular systems

Beginners – Follow the sequence from positions 1 – 3 only.

Intermediate – PLOW: From the final raised position in SHOULDER STAND, bring the legs forward and begin to lower the feet until they are above and behind the back of the head. The legs remain straight. Slowly release the position of the hands and place the arms on the mat beside the body, palms face down.

Lower the legs further directly behind the head, parallel to the mat. The bottom of the toes contact the mat behind the head and the legs remain straight. The chin is retracted, the palms and arms are face down on the mat with the weight of the body in the arms, shoulders, head, and toes. Close the eyes. Maintain the asana for 10 respirations.

Advanced – DEAF MAN: From PLOW, slowly bend and drop the knees beside the ears. Rotate the arms around and grasp the ankles. The top of the feet and shins rest on the mat. The gluteals are in the air and the body weight rests in the shoulders, head, and feet. Close the eyes. Maintain the asana for 10 respirations.

CONTRA-INDICATIONS

Do not practice this asana if experiencing: low back injuries, sciatica, spinal pathologies, neck trauma, symptoms of whiplash, spinal osteoporosis, cardio vascular disease, or in the advanced stages of pregnancy.

PRECAUTION

Keep the neck straight. Do NOT turn the head from side to side. This may cause severe damage.

Navasana – the boat Pose

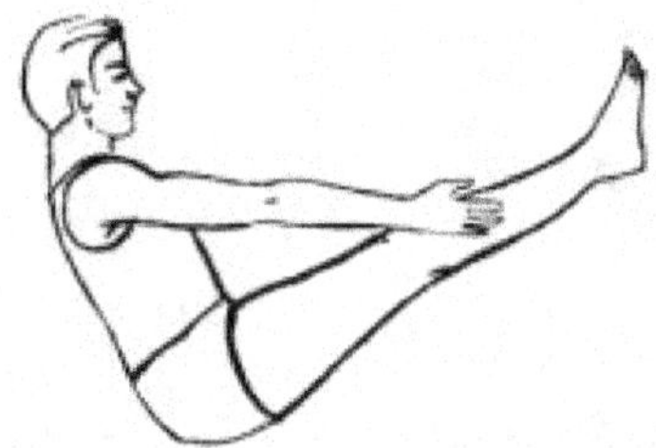

Benefits: Strengthens your abdominal muscles, and your sense of self and willpower. Builds up your core strengths

How to do –

Sit up with the soles of your feet flat on the floor.

Hook your hands behind your hamstrings and lean back slowly until you are balancing up on your sit bones.

Lift your feet off of the ground and, with bent knees, raise your feet up, so they are aligned with your knees.

Press your lower back in and extend your chest up to the sky. Release your hands from behind your hamstrings and reach your arms out in front of you, palms facing together.

Make sure you keep pressing your shoulders down, pressing your lower back in and extending your heart up. Hold the pose for 5 breaths.

Advanced practitioners can extend their legs straight, making a "V" shape.

How to do Sukh Padam Asana

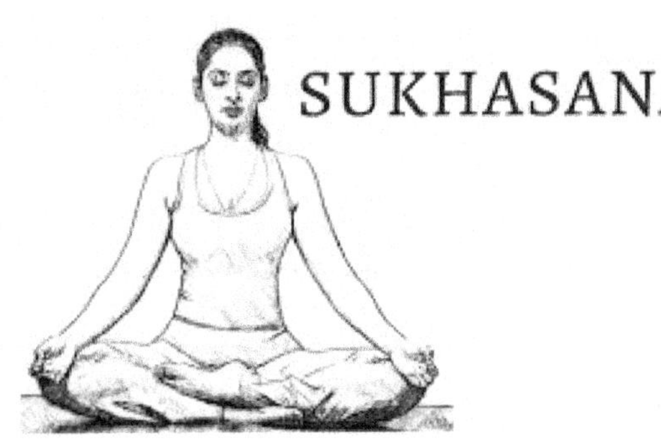

Benefits

• Stabilizes the pelvis and hips

• Increases breath capacity

• Elongates the spine from the sacrum to the base of the skull

• Facilitates mental and physical balance

Intermediate – HALF LOTUS: Sit upright with the legs straight in front of the body. Bend the right leg and place the bottom of the right foot against the inner left thigh. Bend the left leg and place the left foot on top of the right thigh. Without straining, try to place the upper heel close to the abdomen. Lift the sternum, retract the shoulder blades, and engage the core.

Place the hands on the knees, palms face up. Inhale, lengthen the neck, retract the chin, and lift the crown of the head. Draw the shoulder blades further down, and expand and lift the rib cage. Gaze at the eyebrow center or close the eyes. Maintain the asana for 10 respirations. Repeat on the other side.

Advanced – LOTUS: Sit upright with the legs straight in front of the body. Slowly and gently bend the right leg and place the right foot on top of the left thigh. The bottom of the right foot faces upward and the heel is close to the pubic bone.

Bend the left leg and place the left foot on top of the right thigh. Without straining, place the upper heel close to the abdomen. In the ideal position both knees eventually touch the mat. Lift the sternum, retract the shoulder blades, and engage the core.

Place the hands on the knees, palms face up. Inhale, lengthen the neck, retract the chin, and lift the crown of the head. Draw the shoulder blades further down, and expand and lift the rib cage. Gaze at the eyebrow center or close the eyes. Maintain the asana for 20 respirations. Repeat on the other side.

Contradictions

Do not practice this asana if experiencing: hip, knee, or ankle problems; sciatica; low back complications; or injuries.

Basic principles of Mula Bandha

In yoga there are three classic areas of focused potential and dormant energy in the human body: Pelvis – Mula Solar – Uddiyana Throat – Jalandhara The pelvic or mula region is the most powerful of the three areas where there is an abundance of potential energy. This energy is generally scattered and used intermittently for sexual acts. Asana practice is a wonderful way to cultivate and use this energy for physical strength and mental clarity. The powerful technique used to awaken and direct this energy is called the Mula Bandha.

The word 'bandha' is defined as 'a seal' – to seal within, interconnect the inner systems. The bandhas are engaged physically, but their effects are on the overall energy and awareness levels of the mind. The Mula Bandha used in yoga asanas has many benefits. The Mula Bandha works synergistically. Engaging the 'core lock' enables the asanas to be held longer, protecting the low back muscles, making the practice of asanas safer. When the Mula Bandha is fully engaged, dormant potential energy is activated into the conscious network resulting in more support in the core lock. The distal muscle groups relax drawing the body energy levels from the periphery to the center.

MULA BANDHA
THE ROOT LOCK - FOR WOMEN

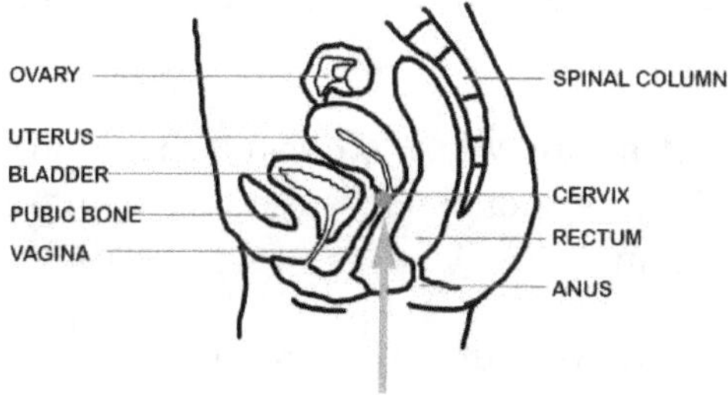

CONTRACT THE SPOT NEAR THE CERVIX

Females engage the Mula Bandha by exhaling, contracting the muscles between the pubic bone and the tailbone, and lightly drawing the perineum up and in toward the abdomen. Pull the pelvic floor up toward the spine and feel the lower, deep abdominal muscles engage.

Initially the anus and genitals need to be contracted, but with practice over time these areas become relaxed and the contraction is isolated to the perineum (the space between the anus and genitals). Specifically draw the opening of the cervix up and in.

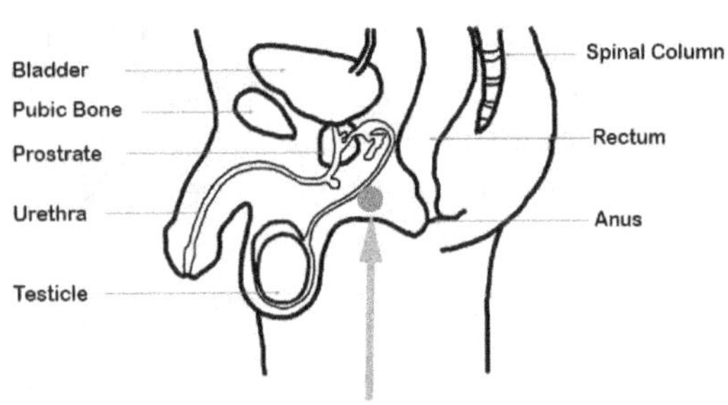

Males engage the Mula Bandha by lifting up the space an inch above the perineum, forming a triangle. The perineal space becomes indented, domed, and sucked in and up, creating empty space for the front of the pubic bone and sacrum to move toward each other.

The intensity of the Mula Bandha contraction can be carried from 15 – 100 percent and it may be held for as long as possible.

Mental and health benefits of yoga – Fighting Corona and other Diseases

Yoga keeps not only the body but also the mind healthy.By doing yoga,Dhyan & Prananayan we can keep our mental & health benefits.In these days of lockdown when it is not possible to go out there is a feeling of boredom and frustrations sitting at home.Sometimes this results in fear of unknown,worry and depression.

By doing yoga we can be internally and externally strong.Let us know how we can remain in mental balance and healthy while staying in home in lockdown period.We should not fear it but to put ourself safe by staying at home and do yoga asanas,dhyan and pranayam.

According to Maharishi Patanjali formula : yogashata dissolves power but liberation is possible,removes inherent occupied tensions but keeps mind in control.

By following some asans we can keep our body healthy and mind in a happy and joyful state.Yogasana removes stress and negativity contributing mind to be a calming place.We can follow Pranayam and Yognidra for this.

Benefits of Pranayam

In yoga breath is called Pranavayu.The correct method of taking and controlling breath is called Pranayam.By focusing on our breath we can control negative emotions that is the root of stress.Kapalbhatti,Bhastrika,Nadi shodhan,Bhramri and Surya Namaskar reduces stress,tension and depression and keeps us healthy.

Remember Yogasana and pranayam should be done in empty stomach or four to five hours after taking a meal.Als wear comfortable clothes while practicing yoga asanas.

Benefits of Yoga Nidra

After doing yoga asana the next step is to do yoga nidra for some period.Practising Yognidra helps in calming mind and making it afresh.Yoga sleep increases concentration and memory sharp.It also helps in cleansing harmful chemicals from our body.

Remember If by doing some asana if there is feeling of uneasiness or pain it is advisable to not do that asana for it may cause problem.

Some other Asana like Dhanursana, shirshasana,Siddhasana are also beneficial to increase immunity and benefit mental and physical health.

Benefits of Dhanurasana

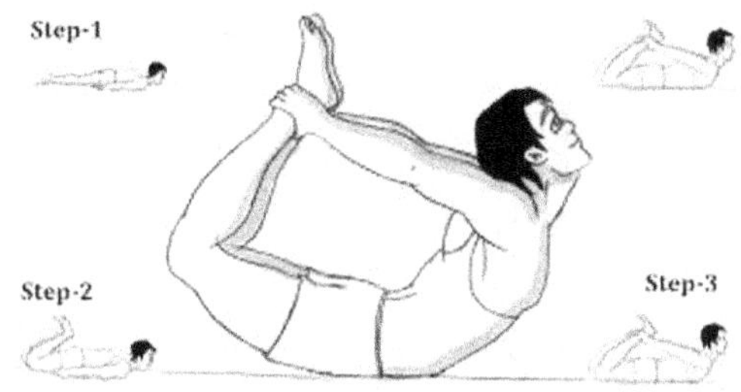

Dhanurasana is consisted of 2 words: Dhanu means that 'bow' and posture indicates a Yoga pose. therefore the name is 'the Bow Pose' as a result of within the final position, the body resembles a bow.During this cause, the abdomen and thigh representing the picket a part of the bow whereas legs lower elements and arms representing the cord.

The way to Dhanurasana Yoga

How to perform Dhanurasana may be a terribly easy procedure. the various techniques and steps of doing the Bow cause ar being given below:

Steps for Dhanurasana

First of all change posture in prone position

Exhale, bend your knees and hold the ankles with hands

While inhaling raise the thighs, head and chest as high as you could.

Try to maintain weight of the body on lower abdomen. Now join the ankles. Look upward and breathe easily.

While breathing , bring down the head and legs up to knee. Maintain this position as long as you'll hold and slowly return to the initial position.

Benefits of Shirshasana

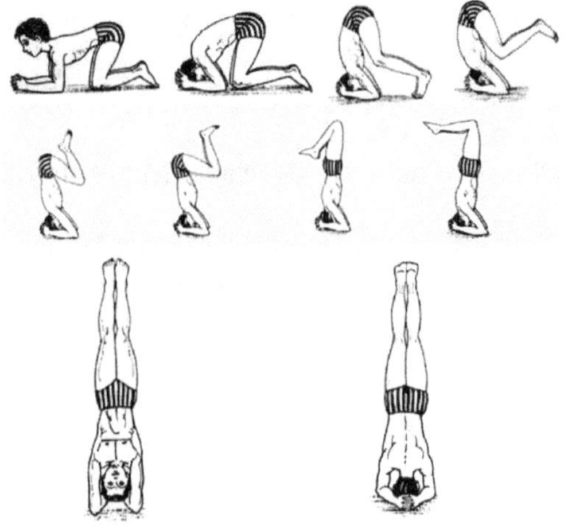

The shirshasana is also one such asana which is done on the head. Shirshasana is considered to be the best among yogasanas. The shirshasana is also known as Vriksasana and Kapalasana. There are many benefits of shirshasanas that is why it is considered very useful. But it is also important to know what is the head position, what are its benefits. How the shirshasana is done. Which people should not do shirshasana.

To know all these things, one has to know what the head position is. Let us know what the head position is.

Process of shirshasana

The shirshasana should be done on a sheet or blanket.

For this you should choose a flat place.

For shirshasana, first of all you should sit in Vajrasana. You sit in such a way that you have enough space to lean forward.

Sitting in Vajrasana, join the fingers of both hands together by resting both elbows on the ground.

Your palms should be upwards by joining the fingers of both hands, so that you can support the palms of your head.

Slowly bending forward, keep your head on the palms and keep the breath normal. Then slowly let the body load on your head.

In this position, you have to lift your legs towards the sky, just as you stand on the feet straight, in the same way you are standing upside down.

Stay in this position for some time and then come back to normal.

Benefits of Siddhasana

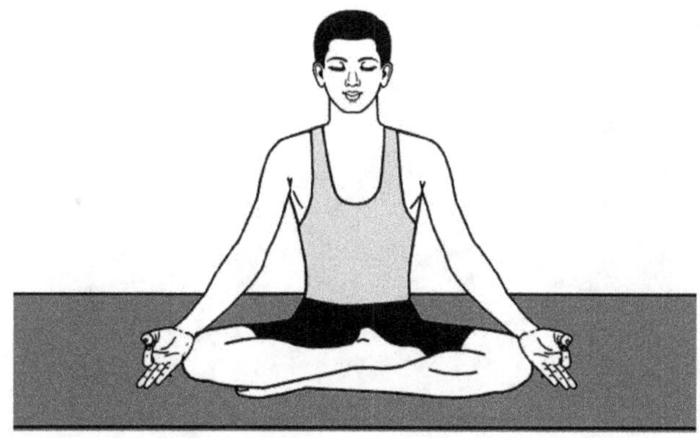

Siddhasana described in yoga is a meditative yogasana. It is known as the best posture among all yogasanas. It provides countless siddhis and suppressing diseases, due to which it is known as Siddhasana.

Commonly practiced by the practitioner during meditation or other compound actions. These asanas help in awakening the Kundalini by making the life upward.

How to do Siddhasana

Siddhasana should be practiced in a quiet place. So that you can easily connect with yourself, and stabilize the mind.

First of all sit in Dandasana (with legs spread in front) by laying mat on the ground.

Keep the waist straight.

Fold the left leg from the knee and place the heel between the anus and testicles.

While doing this, close the soles of the left foot with the thigh of your right foot.

Now bend the right foot from the knee and press the heel over the penis.

While doing this, keep the soles of the right foot adjacent to the inner part of the left thigh.

Place both hands on the knees (you can keep your hands in any posture). Keep the spine, chest and neck upright and apply Jalandhar Bandha.

Focus your attention for some time between the Bhrkuti.

Come back to normal after some time.

Repeat the above action by changing the legs.

Defeat Corona with Yoga - Quit Smoking

It's been days of lockdown due to the intention of breaking the chain of viruses.Now Laxman Rekha has drawn,so there is a lot of benefit at this time to quit bad habits indeed the cycle of smoking chain by embracing yoga and keep our life secure and safe.With yoga,pranayam and meditation we can feel the supreme bliss that is called the "state of Ananda".Of course this is the best time to thank God for the world, life he created.He lifts you to such a great height that any desire of bad habits dies within you internally.

The days of terror of Corona Virus infection.The authentic report states that Corona Virus deteriorate the Health of your lungs.Its the first to attack the respiratory system and spoils it. Reports Coming from all over the world suggest that the cause of Corona Virus the most people who have died have lungs infected.Had a disease. Actually Corona Virus attacks the lungs and thickens the muscles causing the person to have trouble in breathing.

The condition of the lungs is also very delicate. And also that the corona virus in such a situation,directly access to this weak link.There are few asanas to do that re strengthens your weak detroited lungs from smoking and other bad habits.Asanas that can increase your immunity,increase your mental level as of now to which you have to take the help of nicotine.

Generally doing yoga and meditation to get help to quit smoking we get mainly five types of benefits –

1The body becomes strong. New life in lungs Is filled.

2. The immune system starts getting better.

3. The level of health starts improving.

4. Brain becomes calm and stable.

5. We are full of energy and life force

It is said that if someone does something for consecutive days, then it becomes his habit.Now it is a period of lock down then your bad addiction like smoking can be beneficial to be stopped and finished. So for your smoke.You might have tried to quit the habit, but instinctively have finally broke this vow. Now when availability of nasal products completely closed,in this way, it is a golden gift of your life.New this icing can be made for you.Believe there are many such postures.

With Pranayama and Meditation you can feel the pleasure. Of course, the god has given you the last chance to quit this habit.Surely smoking is an invitation for the attack to Corona Virus that is damaging your respiratory system. Even if your resolve is still shaking make sure that you keep this in mind,an infection that has no cure Inviting for two puffs,It is suicide. Why should we all go to lock down.

Is sitting at home not only to save life ? In this situation how alarming to think of Corona.Those who fear are not worried about cancer? So enough now, break with this toxic smoke and prepare the lungs with the help of yoga.For a positive and healthy life so that someone Corona, never let any cancer weaken you.Could help your loved ones indeed.

Here are some of the yoga practices that can help to increase your immunity to fight against Corona Virus and quit smoking helping you in developing a more refined human being in this age.

Note – According to WHO report 60 lac people die from smoking.From this figure 50 lac people directly die due to active smoking while 10 lac from passive smoking.Nearly more than 4000 chemicals gets inside our body due to smoking.Out of which almost 50 becomes the reason for occurence of deadly Cancer.

Kapalbhati Exercise

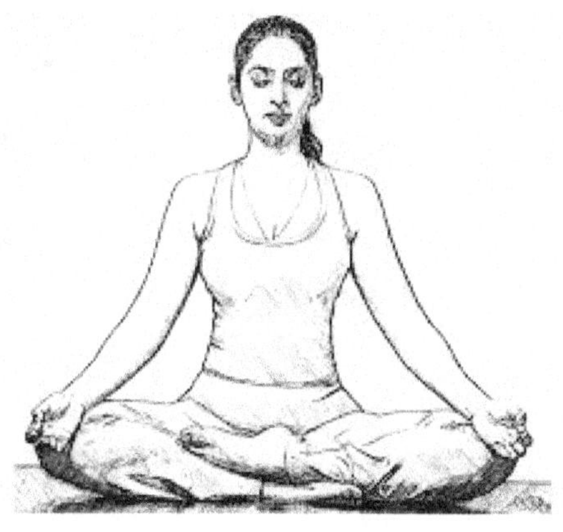

Importance of Kapalbhati

Improvement In blood circulation

Energy to nervous system

Strengthing brain cells and makes it calm

keeps the pulse under control and Control desire

Nadi shodhan Pranayam

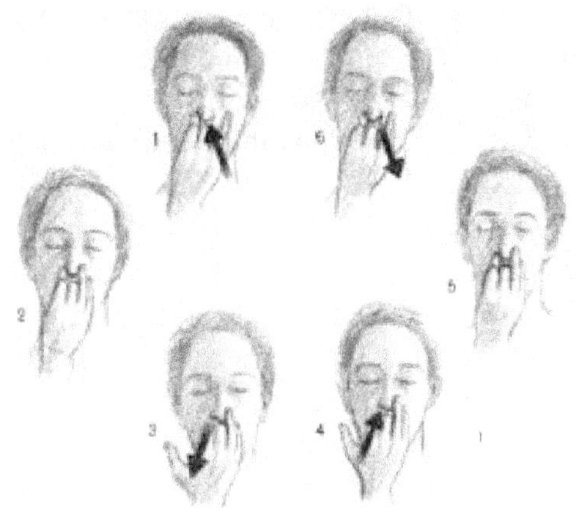

Importance of Pranayam

Removes all types of stress.

keeps the mind calm.

Calms and balances the pulse.

Therapeutically resolves all respiratory problems

To help from overcoming any kind stress while stopping bad habits.

Trikonasana

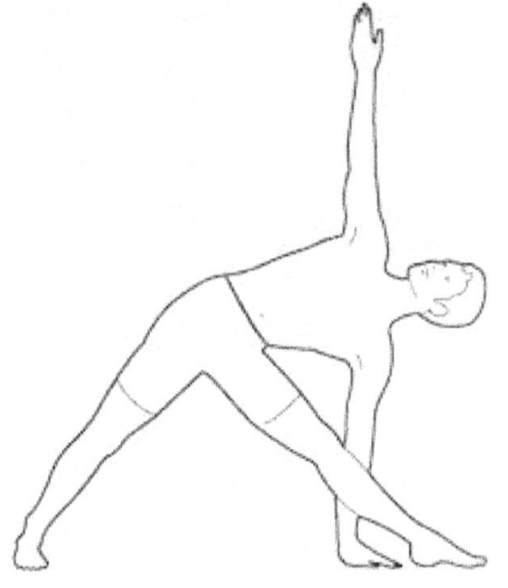

Benefits of Trikonasana

Creates good stretch in different parts of the body.

Helps in physical and mental health

Helps the desire to quit smoking

Creates flexibility and strength

Bhujangasana

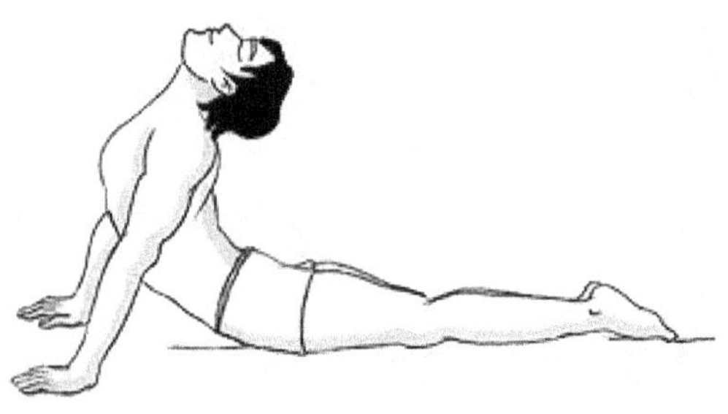

Benefits of Bhujangasana

It Increases chest Size

Improves circulation of blood

Helps people from nasal related problems

Setuband asana

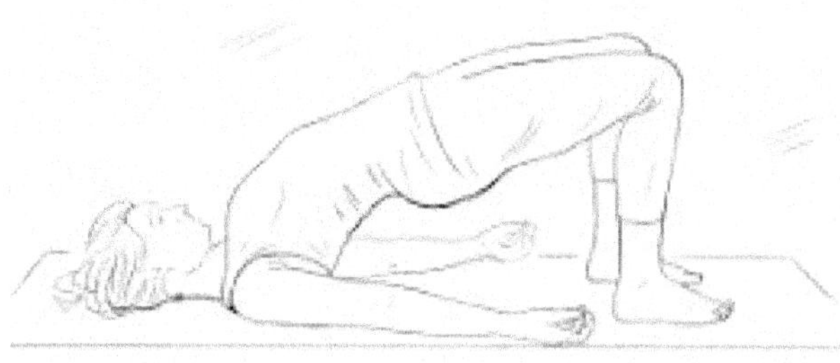

Benefits of Setuband asana

Helps to open lungs.Stimulates in proper oxygen flow

Maintains in stretching of various parts of body

Keeps mind cool and calm

Helps to reduce stress,tension and depression
Helps to quit smoking

Sarvangasana

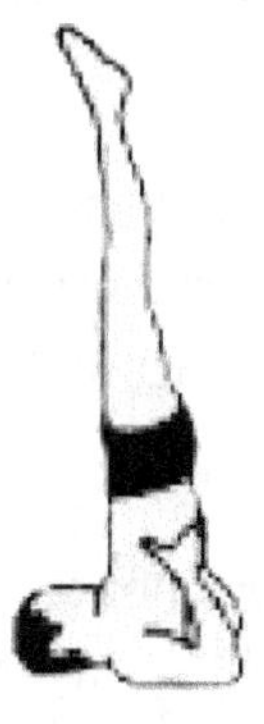

Benefits of Sarvangasana

Helps in proper blood circulation simultaneously development of mind

Keeps mind in calming position

Controls depression and stress that helps to stop the desire for smoking.

Yoga benefits for the kids

We love Yoga and knows its benefits.So why not get the children involved and share the benefit with them too.This will be a great help for their development.

Our children today have very busy lives running at school and sports commitments, busy parents, video games and lightning speed among many other stimuli. We do not usually think that these are stressful for our children, but in many cases they are, and these stresses can negatively impact their innate pleasure.

Just as you find yoga helpful to release your stresses, similarly children too, so why not take it home? Your combined yoga experience can have a lot of benefits, not only because of the change in your children, but through the change it will create in your perspective!

The 7 main benefits of yoga for children are:

Increases concentration - As children learn various yoga positions, and learn to control their body through these positions, they develop their self-control and increase their focus

Sparks Creativity and Imagination - If you encourage your children to make a dog-like noise in a dog pose and whisper like a snake in a cobra pose, and encourage them to imagine that they are the character of the pose , You make them great imagination

Increase body awareness - Different poses of yoga help children to listen to their body, which is an invaluable tool for life.

Increases self-esteem - As their focus, flexibility and their techniques improve, it will increase your child's self-esteem.

The present moment teaches awareness - as their mind has to focus on their breathing and technique, it stops them thinking about the future or living in the past

Provides tools for stress management - Yoga provides an immediate outlet for stress and creates pleasurable endorphins

Discipline and responsibility teaches - As yoga is a process, by practicing regularly they learn that it is a process that is not an immediate destination and through this they can accept that life is a path.

To reap the benefits of yoga for children, you must translate it into their language to give both you and your children a better experience. You need to learn to hold their attention for a long time to teach them the benefits of meditation, balance, flexibility, meditation, peace, health and well-being.

Children get a chance to pretend animals, trees and warriors. Sound is also a great outlet for them, so encourage them to let the sounds come out while practicing each situation.

Sharing yoga as a family has a great power to strengthen the family and due to its adaptable nature you can be more flexible about the moment of yoga. You do not need to go outside for 30 minutes to do yoga on children, you can incorporate simple stretches and breathing exercises for any time of the day.

You will find that your yoga moments will help to create fun, build confidence, engage in teamwork and deepen the family body.

As you can see there are many benefits of teaching yoga to your children, not only for them but also for you, so why not try it today and enjoy and enjoy your yoga moments.

Yoga Stories of fun Can Benefit Your Child

As a parent you have to be careful about what you are teaching your child. Children are friendly and eager to learn and if you give them the right kind of education and environment, they will grow up to become self-sufficient people.

Education today is far from imparting bookish knowledge, it has to be holistic in its true sense of the word and still be simple enough for young children to enjoy the learning process.

A great educational tool to teach children

Using yoga can be a great educational tool for parent.Your children need exercise and yet have a child who does not love stories, so why not mix the benefits of both? Yoga stories will not only help your children improve their health and resilience, but it will also spark their curious imaginations.

Today there are many certified yoga trainers who specialize in children's yoga who say that such stories are very beneficial for children between two and eight years of age.

Yoga stories are constructed in a way to encourage children to move forward while having fun and learning all the way. Yoga stories can be practiced in many creative ways. Let us illustrate with an example that can be used on children or young children between the ages of 3-5.

Find a big bag and put all kinds of stuffed toy animals in them. You can then talk to each child about the trip to the zoo and weave it into the story format.

Each child gets a toy to pick up the animal and mimic its pose. A yoga expert who has to oversee this activity will see that the child performs each pose correctly. Before you know it you will find that the children are acting out the story and making their fantasies wild!

There are many yoga places that organize special events like the ones mentioned above. Stories like these teach young minds not only about animals, but about different people, places and cultures.

Develops a child's physical and creative abilities

In this way learning yoga in a constructive way will help children to develop awareness of their body and improve their skills.The focus of this innovative way of learning is not to teach children about correct yoga postures,it is about promoting an attitude of kindness and gratitude. Through such programs children learn the benefits of sharing, collaboration and acceptance.

It has been observed that children who learn through yoga stories are able to build their strength and flexibility over time.These children are less prone to throw tantrums and develop a sense of self-expression as well as being relaxed and calm.

If you are a parent who is encouraging your children to learn through yoga stories, do not pressure your children to focus on things like learning the right posture or losing weight. You should just encourage them to have fun in the best way.

Benefits of Yoga for the Youth

Youth is a state at which time there is maximum vigor, enthusiasm and enthusiasm. Hard work and struggle are most common in this stage. There are many desires and desires in this state.

If you use the energy of young age in the right direction, then it is beneficial with your growing age. Because as the age increases the body becomes weak, irritability in the mind and decrease in the body's elation.

It is important that you focus your mind in your youth and increase your concentration. Also, make the body healthy so that you will be able to face the coming challenges.

You can store your energy by meditating and make your dreams come true in your youth. Know which are Meditation Mantras for Youth.Elders do yoga, but they only worry about health and they also do convenient yoga. The whole world is lying in front of the youth.

Why Yoga for Youth is necessary

We are mentally and physically healthy. We will take away this freshness from nature, because it is our right. Now the question arises why do yoga again. Hey brother, had to learn meditation and yoga before archery, because with that, warriors could become proficient in weapons and weapons. After meditation, the arrow will hit the right target in one go... Got it. There were some wars which used to discourage the goal from their thinking! Why work hard to shoot undeserved arrows?

In the Buddhist period, monks had to learn such disciplines as yoga, martial arts and judo karate. You would think that if monks should deal with meditation and meditation, then this is not the case. Earlier forests and wild animals and wild humans were dangerous. The earlier natural outbreaks were no less terrible.

The saints of the past used to be more dangerous than the warriors, only then they used the power to catch a big thing like salvation by swooping like an eagle. Moksha is not a game of children and elders, understand. In the same way, in today's modern life, new types of wild have become man-made, now the need for yoga has increased, otherwise you too may wait to grow old and die.

Yoga format for youth

When we say 'yoga' it does not mean just asana. Yoga is the name of the complete types of Yama, Niyam, Asana, Pranayama, Pratyahara, Dharana, Dhyana and Samadhi. Choose two types from the first five above. Anyway, it would be better if you make your own format. Yoga says that following is another suicide. Yes, it can be advised here that the beginning should be done by organ operation.

Benefits of yoga for youth

Increase level of confidence

The first thing is to ask yourself this question. Know what your problem is. The answer will come out automatically. To be young and to look, one has to do yoga. How long will the other dimensions of fake confidence, health, or ability gained from the twelve last. If a lion will stand in front of you, how will you look in his eyes and talk? In English, PD class or management class, how much confidence will be extended by screaming. Can you stand on the tip of the peak of the mountain where the strong wind blows? What will you do when a mountain of sorrow falls in life?

Make your dreams come true

Every youth has his or her own desires and aspirations, which he wants to fulfill.It is possible through meditation. Meditation increases confidence and concentration.By meditating regularly, youth can make their wishes come true.

Be friendly to everyone

Nature makes a big difference in youth.The temperament is fickle at a young age which needs to be centered.Meditation is a medium through which you can control your mind with regular practice and make it suitable for the environment.If your nature becomes favorable then you will also be humble towards others and you will also be able to become many friends.

Gaining Stability

Youth is a state in which we have to face many situations from which we run.Due to these problems we are surrounded by stress and anxiety.If you meditate daily, then you will be able to stay away from this anxiety and stress and this will also increase the self-confidence.

Be in love with parents

In young age, the tendency is agitated and irritable, due to which we are not able to speak properly to our family members, especially the parents.Meditation keeps your mind calm, it develops your thinking power, so that you are able to talk peacefully with your mother and father.Because meditation makes you smarter and develops the power of understanding in you.

Direct your energy

The youth is full of energy, vigor, enthusiasm and enthusiasm.The correct development of this energy is done through meditation, which works to make this energy creative and active.

Power of Meditation

There are many benefits of meditating daily.It helps in keeping the body healthy.There are many bad habits which do not remain for life in youth. Meditation can also help you for this.Meditation increases focus and accuracy.

Think out of the box

Everyone feels that he is the most out of it.Through meditation, you develop the power to think in a new way and you become creative.

Yoga for Removing Toxins from the Body

We always want peace and balance in our mind and body.The only way we can achieve this is through detoxification i.e removing toxins from body.As you move forward in life, your body accumulates some toxins that are slowly formed.

These toxins have some devastating health effects.They have some negative effect on the clarity of our mind and this also reduces our energy level.When you detoxify, it will help you deal with all these negative symptoms.

There are various ways that one can detoxify his or her body system.It is very important for you to do deep research, which is perfect for you.One of the safest ways you can detoxify the body is by consuming a whole fruit which is a plant-based diet.

In fact, consume more vegetables and reduce animal products as well as processed foods. A lot of fruits and vegetables contain some nutrients as well as micronutrients that allow the body to naturally cleanse itself.

As a matter of fact, consumption of raw fruits and vegetables should be encouraged to achieve maximum cleaning benefits.However,one of the most effective ways to detox the body is through juice cleansing.

Juice cleanses are excellent because they cause the body to absorb nutrients faster and more efficiently, due to the fact that most of the fiber is removed.

If you consider it after eating something,then your body naturally tends to eliminate fiber.To get maximum results, try to consume juice made from fresh organic products.

How Detox Yoga Helps Facilitate Cleansing

Most vigorous forms of exercise help to stimulate all three systems of elimination to some extent, helping to cleanse the body as well as detox.

Yoga and its focus is on organizing every part of the body as well as systematically spreading,especially being well suited to keeping the body's waste removal channels in a state that it can function properly.

In a well-rounded yoga practice, every part of your body is involved.This is because you have to push, pull, jerk your body, as well as bend your body.

This will help speed up the removal of waste products such as; Carbon dioxide,lactic acid as well as lymphatic fluid gets buried in the deep tissues and ends of the body that cannot even jog or ride a bike.

Detoxification best trick and measure

Pranayama is the source of freshness in yoga

Pranayama is made up of two words – 'Pran' and 'Ayam'. 'Prana' means life or age and 'ayam' means length. So Pranayama simply indicates long life. The yogic practice that increases the duration of life is called Yogic Pranayama. According to Maharishi Patanjali, "Pranayama is the ability to control Prana".

Prana is the power of consciousness which is present in the entire universe including the human body.Prana controls the brain and senses.According to Ayurveda,Prana is different from Vayu. It is the prana that carries the air into the body through the "panch prana".

Prana: Prana carries air from mouth to nasal to heart. This causes breathing.

Saman: It carries air from the heart to the navel and performs subtle activities.

Apan: It moves air from the navel to the feet and performs the function of urination and excretion.

Udaan: It carries air from the throat towards the head and keeps it in an upright position.

Vyan: It is present throughout the body.

Pran does his work in a sequence as shown:

- Rechak: to exhale breath
- Poorak: to breathe in
- Kumbhak: Hold the breath
- Bahay Kumbhak: To Breathe And Stop
- External Kumbhak: exhaling and stopping breath
- Kaivalya Kumbhak: Just to stop the breath (whatever it is)

Yogic Pranayama: The continuous practice of pranayama by yogis is called yogic pranayama.

Preparation before doing yoga pranayama:

1. Yogic "Shat Kriya"
2. Follow celibacy
3. Perfection in yoga pranayama
4. Regularity
5. Concentration of mind
6. The ratio of poor, kumbhak and laxative should be 1: 4: 2 and for beginners it should be 1: 2: 2.
7. Pranayama should be accompanied by all three 'bandhs' wherever applicable.
8. The purak and Rechak should be accompanied by a mool bandh and udyan bandh.
9. Mool Bandh and Jalandhar should be with Kumbhak.
10. Meditation and Mantra with Pranayama

11. Poorak should be done twice of Rechak
12. Pranayama can be done three times a day in the evening, morning and afternoon.
13. If one does not have the proper knowledge to do yoga pranayama, one should do so under expert guidance.

Method of doing yogic pranayama:

1. Sit in Padmasana. Exhale as much as you can. It is known as Rechak.
2. Now pull the genitalia and prevent air from entering.Keep this condition up to the threshold.It is called "Bahya Kumbhak".
3. Now inhale while repeating the mantra or Om 'slowly'. It is called poorak.
4. When the lungs are full of air, hold the air. It is known as "Antara Kumbhak".
5. When you feel restless, release the air slowly so that most of the air comes out of the lungs.

Benefits of Pranayama:

1. It cleans the airways and prevents respiratory diseases.
2. It purifies the blood and removes toxins from the body.
3. It gives relief in Vata, Pitta and Kapha diseases.
4. It reduces high blood pressure by normalizing blood pressure.
5. It refreshes the body.

Precaution:

1. Do not do pranayama in dirty environment.
2. It should not be done in strong wind.
3. It should not be done on the bed while covering the face.
4. This should not be done before and after two hours before meals.
5. Although it can be done at any time, the time before sunrise is quite beneficial.
6. Pregnant women and physically weak people should not do this.
7. While doing the poorak, the stomach should be pulled out, while doing it again it should be pulled inside.

Yoga for Weight Loss

Yoga is considered to be a wonderful practice for gaining spiritual knowledge.Yoga is also a great physical exercise for weight loss.Experts say that the physical aspect of hatha yoga or yoga involves specific physical postures or alignment exercises that help a person achieve the physical fitness necessary to attain spiritual enlightenment.Although yoga works on all parts of the body,it is particularly helpful in reducing body fat and fighting obesity i.e yoga for weight loss.As we all know that obesity is one of the most common issues that people experience these days.Due to sedentary lifestyles and unhealthy diets, people are becoming obese and suffering from a severe form of physical illness called obesity.

We tell you the top five yogasanas that can help you fight obesity –

1 Naukasana or Boat Pose

As the name suggests,Naukasana or Boat Pose helps you reduce abdominal fat, tone abdominal muscles and strengthen your lower back.

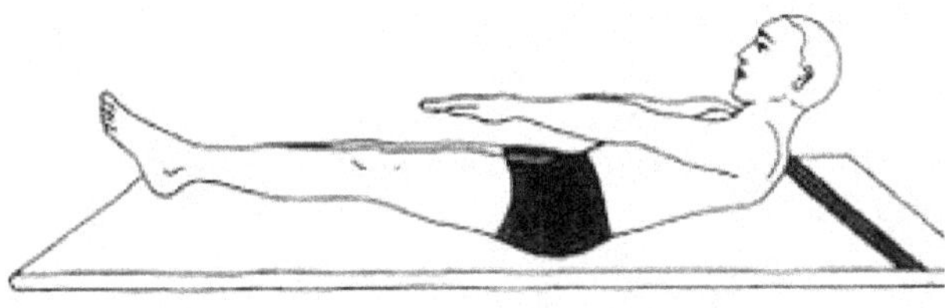

Lie on your back. Keep your hands with your body. Take a few deep breaths. Now slowly take a deep breath, lift your body, chest, hands and feet off the floor.Continue this position for a few seconds or as long as you can. Feel the stretch on your chest, abdomen and back muscles constantly. Slowly return to normal. While exhaling, relax the posture and return to the original position. Repeat the asana at least three times.

2 Pawanmuktasan or gas release pose

This pose is very useful for burning fat in your thighs,hips and abdominal area.

Lie on your back.Now slowly raise your feet and place your hands around your knees. In this position, bring your feet closer to the body.Hold this position for few seconds.Slowly release the pose and bring your head to the floor. Once done,straighten your legs and relax.

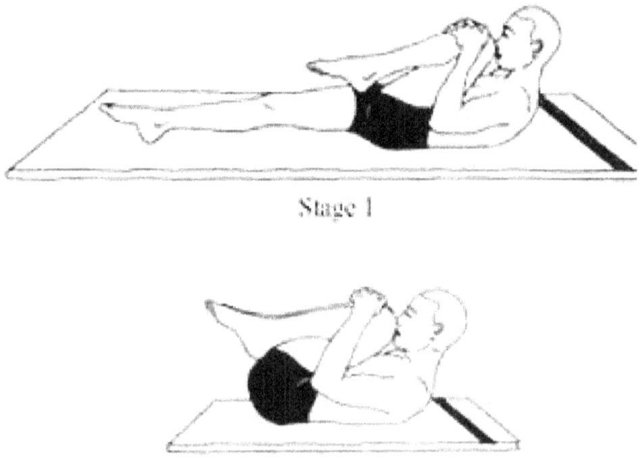

3. Bhujansana or Cobra pose

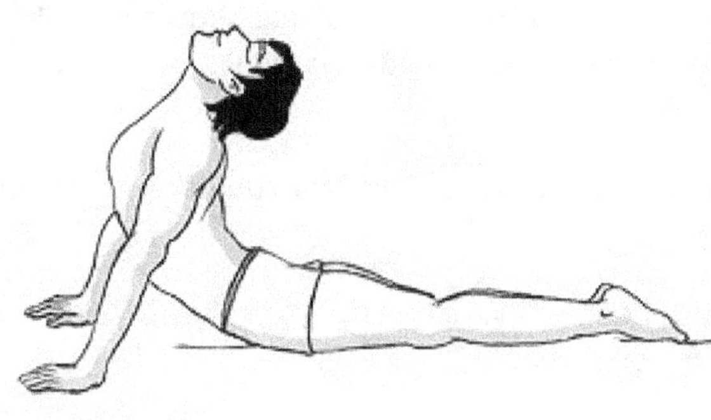

It is also called Cobra pose.This pose is especially helpful in stretching and stretching your arms, shoulders,buttocks, thighs, back and abdomen.Bhujansana is an excellent asana for reducing abdominal fat.If practiced regularly, this pose can help you achieve a flat stomach.

Lie on your stomach on the floor.Place your palms on the ground near the shoulder. Inhale and lift your body up to the navel simultaneously. Hold this pose for a few seconds and slowly return to the original position. Repeat the asana thrice.

4. Paschimottan Asana or forward bend pose

It is considered to be an excellent pose for fighting abdominal fat.This posture helps reduce abdominal fat and tone your abdominal area, pelvic area, thighs,hips,shoulders.

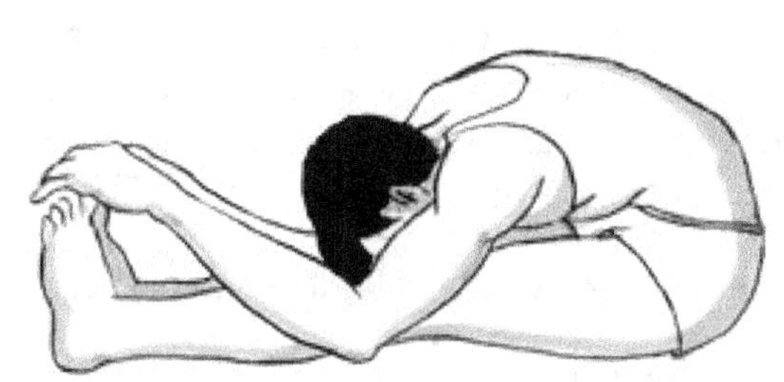

Sit on a flat surface, and spread your legs towards the front and straighten your legs. Inhale and move your arms above your head. Now while exhaling, tilt your body forward and try to touch your knees with your forehead. Continue this pose for a few seconds and keep breathing normally.Inhale and slowly return to normal.Repeat the asana twice.

5. Veerabhadrasan or Warrior-Pose

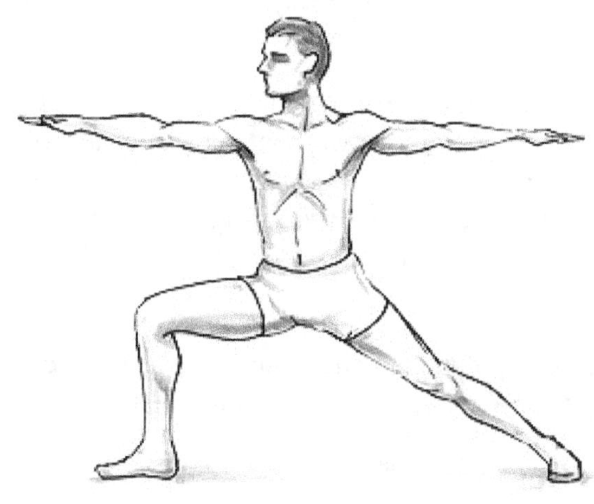

It is also called Warrior Pose.Apart from reducing body fat,this asana also helps to increase body alignment and burn fat throughout the body.

Stand with your feet spread out at least one leg. Now, move your gaze to the right, and bend your right leg at 90 degrees. Now take a deep breath and raise both your arms at shoulder level.Turn your head to the right and continue this pose for a few seconds or as long as you can. Inhale and return to the original position. Repeat the posture at least twice.

Yoga and obesity research

Yoga is one of the techniques used in Ayurvedic medicine to encourage self-healing through the expression of internal and external wells, which can process a potential efficacy to control obesity.

Practicing ancient techniques for the harmony of external and internal body beings through yoga, breath control, meditation,physical movements and gestures known to the people of the Western world and parts of Asia, by various honorable people.The reasons stated are for health related which are approved by the Institutes for Research and Health Advocates.

Obesity is a medical condition of excess body fat accumulation,overweight is a condition of optimum excess body weight, BMI of over 30 is a sign of obesity.

According to Patanjali Yogpeeth, obese patients attended 6 days in which yoga surgery showed a reduction in BMI, fat-free mass and a decrease in total cholesterol.

A total of 47 individuals assessed on the first and last day of the yoga and diet change program, with a 6-day intervention between assessments, showed yoga combination BMI (1.6 percent), waist and hip circumference, fat reduction,total cholesterol (7.7 percent decrease), high-density lipoprotein (HDL) cholesterol (8.7 percent decrease), fasting serum leptin levels (44.2 percent decrease) and increased postural stability and hand grip (P) <0.05, all) comparison).

The study also indicated that intensive yoga programs with changes in diabetes may reduce some of the risks, but the benefits are improved postural stability, grip strength, reduced waist and hip circumference,and reduced learning of serum latines. with. Along with the reduction in levels, there is also loss from obesity.

Determination of yoga learning and participation

In the deed, a non-dimensional, single-arm traditional study was conducted from August 2012 to March 2015 at the Integral Health Clinic, Department of Physiology,All India Institute of Medical Sciences,New Delhi, India insisted that patients who use all types of yoga practice,they not only improved quality of life and health after short-term yoga-based lifestyle interventions,but also demonstrated physical, psychological wells in both male and female subgroups.

These effects include a decrease in body weight,BMI, total body fat, waist and hip circumference,waist-to-hip ratio, fasting glucose in systolic and diastolic blood, total cholesterol, low-density lipoprotein, triglycerides, and fasting glucose in obese participants.

In addition, a chart controller trial with parallel groups (sum and control groups) on 80 male obese with a body mass index (BMI) between 25 and 35 kg / cm2 was divided into two identical groups in which 72 subjects (Yoga n = 37 and control) n = 35) completed the test, after 14 weeks of yoga training with additional yoga practice for the next 3 months, the yoga group had the final result in anthropometric and psychological parameters such as waist, percent body horn, An effective improvement in PSS has been shown.

Overall, obese patients who attended yoga lessons showed a significant change in the control of obesity, of physical and mental well-being, which could lead to weight loss and to reduce complications of obesity.

Benefits of Yoga for Women's Health

Yoga is an ancient art of uniting body, soul and mind.The word yoga denotes unity, communication and integrity in Sanskrit.Yoga originated in ancient India and became popular in the West.Yoga is for all of us,that is a traditional Indian philosophy that unites physical and mental health.With regular practice, we will find that your journey through life is calmer, happier and more fulfilling.Yoga benefits the health of women in the following ways.

Physical pain relief

Nowadays, hypertension is becoming a common serious disease in the world.The practice of yoga can increase blood circulation, bringing blood pressure back to normal.What's more, yoga can help digestion, improve lymph circulation. Yoga also helps cells to get more oxygen. This can reduce heart attacks and strokes as blood clots are often the cause of these diseases.

keeping fit

Yoga is not only a sport, but a healthy lifestyle. It has been proved that this healthy sport can keep women in good shape and keep fit.For women who are suffering from sleep disorder,yoga can help in getting a high quality sleep. Women can also reduce or reduce gynecological diseases. Relaxed exercise can make muscles stronger, improve blood circulation, increase oxygen and nutritional supplies. A few minutes of yoga daily provides the secret to feeling fresh and energetic even after a long time.

Removes pressure

Scientists found that yoga has been associated with improved levels of happiness and improved immune function. This type of sport can help people cope with stress. Business women have to work with computers all day or walk in crowded streets with heels. They will give rise to varicose veins, back pain, low quality sexual function and general fatigue. Yoga is a good way to get relief from muscle soreness. After a busy day of work, before going to bed, it is a good habit to dim the lights and light a scented lamp, forget the heavy work and pressure of life in yoga. After that, you will feel fresh and relaxed.

Yoga helping women in Menopause

Throughout the world, a lot of women enter menopause every year. Studies have shown that 85 percent of women have vasomotor flush during menopause. A lot of studies have been done to find out if yoga can really help women suffering from menopause and where all the results are positive.

Yoga,as well as meditation can be helpful in reducing the symptoms of normal menopause, including the frequency as well as the intensity of hot flashes or vasomotor, sleep and mood, muscle and joint pain, Stress as well as disturbances is involved.

Another very important question that people ask is, can yoga be used to replace hormone replacement therapy? Yes of course Hormones, biochemical molecules that help regulate human functions as well as signaling, are secreted into the bloodstream by the body's endocrine glands, and yogis have, for a very long time, shown the relationship between endocrine and esoteric anatomy Noted Yoga asanas are very helpful. They help to stretch as well as squeeze the endocrine glands. Chanting also activates them in some form through vibration and resonance.Mudra helps stimulate the chakras, the energetic correlates of the glands.

The first question is on every woman's mind; Can yoga help reduce menopause? As women go into menopause, which is usually between the ages of 40 as well as 60, their ovaries begin to slow down their estrogen production.The endocrine glands also try to achieve some type of balance. In addition, the pituitary glands can cause more FSH and LH secretion. However, the adrenal, thyroid, as well as other structures will migrate to produce more estrogen. In such situations, the adrenal glands may already be exaggerated, complicating this ongoing balancing act. Its effects include hot flashes, insomnia, anxiety, depression, as well as irritability. Another consequence of this effect is osteopenia, which results in loss of bone density.

A critical review of the entire process suggests that women who are from the western part of the world are more likely to experience these effects. It is somehow directed to the Western diet but another important contributor is stress. Now the question is, how can yoga help? According to some health reports, most of the symptoms of menopause are the result of sympathetic activation or excessive heat. Yoga provides many ways to increase the body's parasitic response. Pranayama like Shitali and many others are very beneficial. Forward Bend also contributes to this situation. It can help calm the adrenal. Standing poses, inversions as well as energizing pranayamas can also help elevate your mood.

Yoga asans for women to practice every day

If you are looking for some great asans for women, then look no further! The following yoga poses for women are highly recommended for performing them. They basically focus on creating some pressure and also pull specific body parts.

SPINAL-FLEX-ROCK-POSE

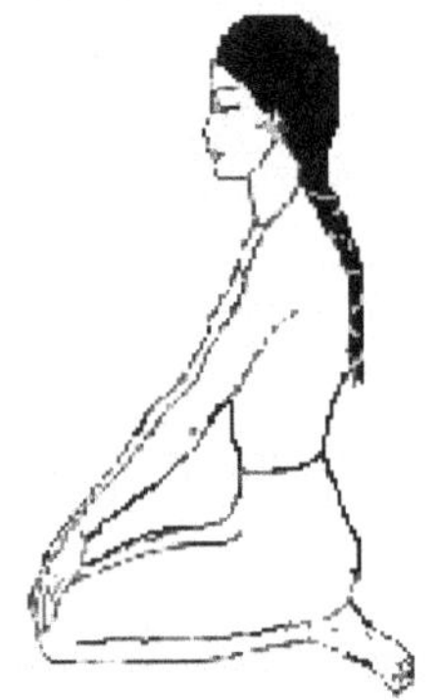

This particular type of yoga posture releases tension in the middle as well as the upper back area.It also helps to move the spinal fluid.This pose is somehow simple.

To practice it, just sit on the heel of your feet.Inhale and tilt the spine forward and at the same time, bring the shoulder blades back.Inhale and push the spine back.

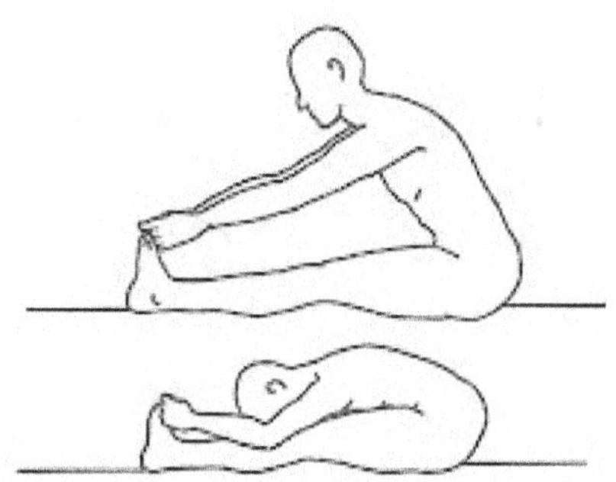

It is an ideal pose to pull the life nerve.It travels from the back of the heel, through the sciatic nerve and over the entire back; It is the lower, middle and upper back.It extends to the neck.

To do this, sit on your right heel and also make sure that the left leg is pushed forward.Tighten the chest to the left and keep it there for some time.Repeat the asana with the other leg.

CAMEL-POSE

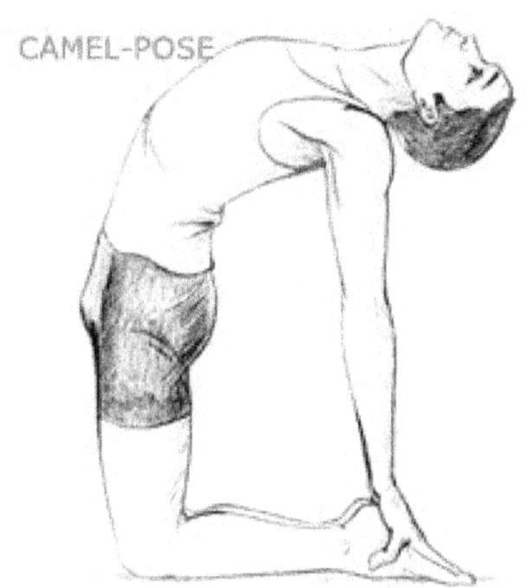

Camel pose is very beneficial for women.It helps in adjusting the reproductive organs of women.To do this, go to your knees and squeeze the gluteus as well.

Also, place your palms backwards which is the kidney area, with the fingers pointing upwards.The next thing you have to do is to bring the hips forward and drop the head back.

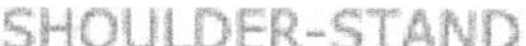

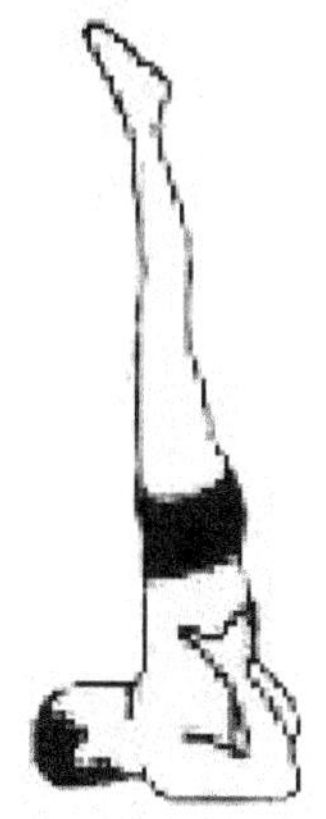

This is another great pose.It helps to stimulate metabolism, which are the thyroid and parathyroid glands.For weight loss, this pose is an excellent one.It also helps release pressure on 11 different organs.

To practice this, just start by lying on your back. Once you have done this, bring your feet above your head, and place your hands on the back for support.Draw as many straight lines as you can between the body and the floor. When performing the action, do not move the neck while looking around. Just gaze at the chest and relax the breath.

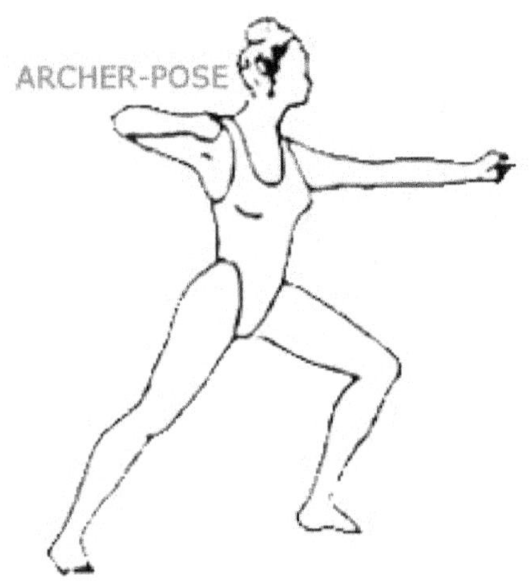

Another excellent pose for women is the archer pose.It helps to stretch the frontal muscles and also opens the hips.To do this, you first have to stand and bring your right leg forward and then bend.

You need to bend it in such a way that it will support the body weight.The left leg should be straight, with the heel off the floor.The right arm also extends forward, as if you are preparing to shoot an arrow. Remember that your hands are in a fist, except the right thumb,which is out and back.

There are many yogas that you can practice, you will benefit from this.The different styles are there to suit your needs as well.Practicing yoga can help eliminate excess fat and maintain your entire body, reducing life and work pressure.From now on, start practicing yoga.

Yoga for Better Sleep

Sleep has an important role in life.Lack of sleep may cause problem in our stability.It is important to do yoga for better sleep.Insomnia is a disease, whose timely treatment is extremely important. But it is not necessary that sleeplessness at night is due to insomnia. Sleep does not occur due to any mental stress or physical fatigue. So you do not have to worry.

Any change in your regular routine or change in direction of sleep or change of location also causes sleeplessness. There are many people who sleep well on their beds. In such a situation, if their place of sleep is changed then they do not sleep all night.

However, after a few days it gets used to it and you start getting better sleep again. If you are also one of those people. If you do not sleep due to small reasons or changes, then you do not need to bother at all.To give you relief from the problem of sleeplessness, here we are telling you some easy yoga.By this practice you will completely remove this problem.

Due to lack of sleep many other diseases surround our body. In such a situation, our body and mind start to ignore any work. It also has an impact on our personal life. In such a situation, you should take help of yoga. This will make you physically and mentally strong, as well as relieve you from the problem of sleeplessness. Know Yoga for Better Sleep –

The practice of these yogasanas will bring good sleep

Udgeeth pranayama

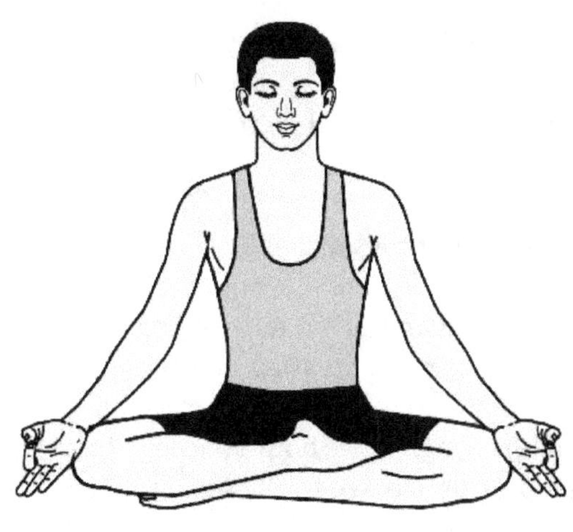

To do this, sit in a state of Padmasana or Sukhasana in a clean and clean environment.

Now take deep long breaths slowly.

After this, chant Om while exhaling breath

Chant 'ॐ' while exhaling for as long as you can.

Breathing has an important role in this pranayama, so keep your full attention on your breath.

While doing this, bring positive thoughts in with the breath and leave negative thoughts out with the breath.

This is a very important pranayama for Yoga for Deep Sleep.

Viparita Karani -The Legs Up The Wall pose

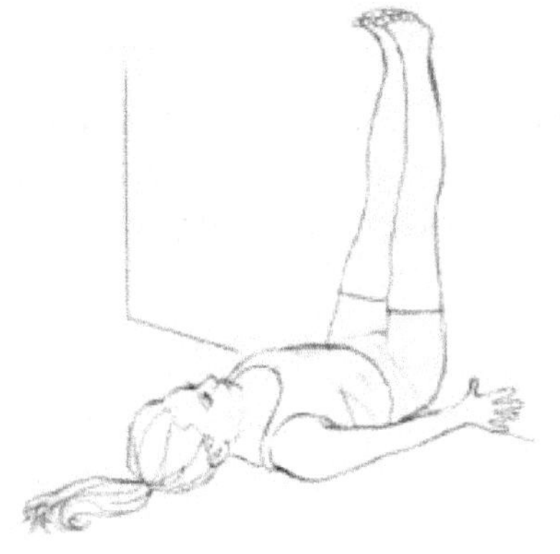

Laying on the mat or yoga mat wall on flat ground, lie on your back and keep your hands straight.

In this case, the hands and feet should be towards the wall.

Now slowly lift the legs and upwards and attach it to the wall.

In the beginning, you can support the hands while raising the back.

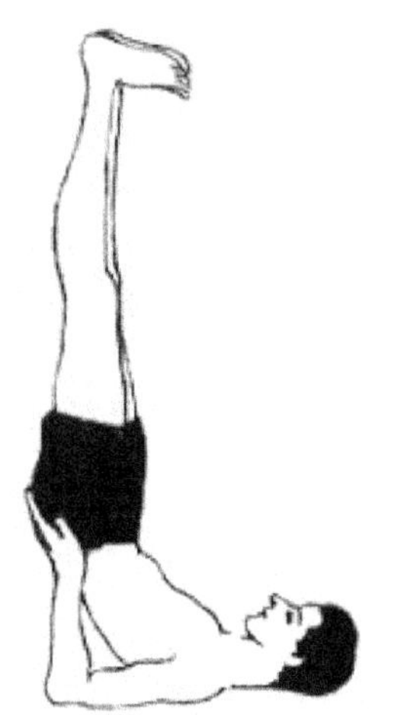

Make sure the elbows are sticking to the ground and the palms support the waist.

In this position your back should be 45 degrees from the ground.

Now take normal breath according to your ability and stay in this posture.

After this, slowly come back to normal.

Butterfly Posture | Butterfly Pose

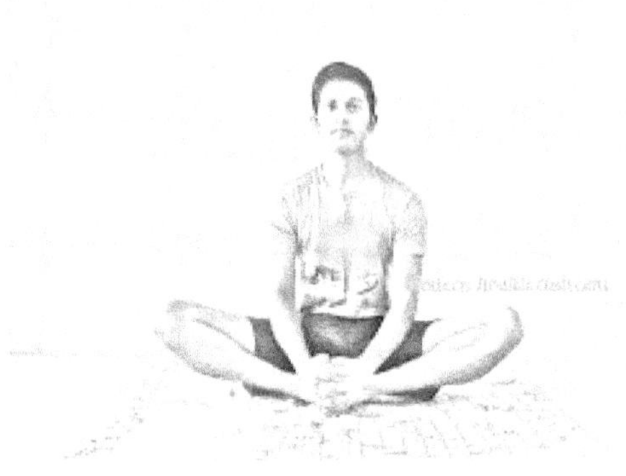

To do this, sit on the ground with the feet facing forward.

After this, hold both your toes by hand.

Now bring the legs near the body, bending from the knee and take long and deep breaths.

In this position, exhaling, move both your legs from the side of the hip upwards like a butterfly's wing.

Make it regular practice as per your ability

It is very beneficial for Yoga for Good Sleep.

It is very easy to keep the body healthy through yoga. This is possible when we practice it correctly. By regularizing Pranayama and Yogasan, you can get relief from the problem of sleeplessness.

Yoga way to stay fit while at work

A consistent fitness routine is the best way to keep your body in good physical shape and your mind healthy.Being active does not mean that you need to spend many hours in the gym.

Doing the things you love, such as walking in the rain, swimming and spending time with loved ones in the forest is the best way to exercise.You can also find ways to fit in some essential work activities, such as taking the stairs and getting up from your desk to walk a short distance every hour.

A typical employee sits in front of his desk for eight hours or more, answering telephone calls, surfing the Internet, writing office communications, and other desk-bound tasks. Sitting all day increases the likelihood of obesity.

There are risks of having poor posture, muscle cramps, and backache. Stretching and deep breathing techniques on your desk can help keep you free from pain and stress during work.

Stretching is an important and easy way to reduce back pain and neck strain. Maintain a flat posture by adjusting the height of your chair and placing your spine behind your chair. This will keep your back and neck bulging and less likely to turn forward which will cause cramps and headaches.

To activate your chest and shoulders during a long day at work, plunge the chair. Place both hands on the arms of your chair and slowly raise your arms down while straightening your arms.

Take yourself back down and stop when your floor is a few inches from the seat, count 5. 15 times. Avoid both wrists by turning both your wrists in circles 10 times.

For lower body stiffness, try to stretch your lower leg alternately,right and left.Then, sitting in your chair, raise one leg and straighten it, but do not bend your knees, count to three and keep your leg down and hold for several seconds. Do this again with your other leg.

More calories are burned than standing and sitting.Instead of using the phone to talk with your colleagues, go to their desk and talk face to face. Stand and stretch your body to answer phone calls. This will give your body a little rest and will also build a stronger relationship with your colleagues.

Bike for walking or working. If you ride a bus or metro, get off at a few blocks or earlier stops and walk the rest of the way.Walking ten extra minutes a day can help you burn extra calories and make you feel more vibrant.

Climb stairs instead of lifts for stepping towards your fitness goals. Use a pedometer to monitor your physical activity and reminds you to keep going. A pedometer is a small device that counts every step you take.

Bringing in fitness gear will also help. Bring a yoga mat that you can use during your break,or a stretch ball to relax your hands and fingers after using the computer.

You can also do push-ups while waiting. Resistance bands - Stretch cords or tubes that offer weight-like resistance when you pull over them - curl some hands on cabinets or drawers and between functions.

Organize groups running lunchtime with your teammates.Encourage everyone to get regular exercise at work and even at home.Schedule walking meetings, if the weather cooperates, take out your walking meetings.

Having regularly scheduled exercise time with your team is a great way to ensure that you exercise on a consistent basis and will build friendships in a shared activity that you can enjoy weekly.

Keep an eye on your diet, eating habits and food intake. This is the most important thing. No one can exercise for a poor diet. Eating cooked vegetables will give you nutrition and improve your digestion.

A homemade lunch instead of vending machine goodies will save your wallet and trim your waistline. Drink warm water before, during and after your activities to stay hydrated. Every system in your body needs water to avoid energy drain and fatigue.

Avoid long hours in front of the TV at home. Your eyes must be tired due to work on computer and screen. Give your eyes a rest. And fall asleep before 10:00 at night. Resting tomorrow and saving more energy for tomorrow. You may also be able to get up and work before work!

Being active is not difficult. Just keep your body moving. Track your progress and make it easy and fun. You will keep your body fit and also build strong relationships with the people around you. And it will lead you to a life full of joy!

How to integrate yoga into a work

It can be a challenge to fulfill all your activities and obligations, even on ordinary days. When you have various professional and personal responsibilities to attend, you may struggle to fit into everything.

As anxiety increases, it is common to lose your peace. Restore your balance and take care of yourself by incorporating some yoga in your daily work routine.

Be Conscious

An important aspect of yoga involves mindfulness.When you focus on stress and what triggers it, you can help reduce it. For example, if a colleague tries to press your button, what can you do to avoid an interchange with this person.

When you have no choice, center yourself and work on regaining your inner peace. Even concentrating on breathing for just a short period of time can be effective for slowing a racing heart and refreshing an anxious mind.

Desk exercise

Many yoga poses are ideal while you sit at the desk.These actions are not comprehensive or difficult, and if you work in an office with others, they will not draw attention to you.

- Pranayama will help you to center yourself when tension increases. Sit in your chair and focus on connecting from your feet.Position your chin so that it is parallel to the floor and center your shoulders on your hips.

Start breathing calmly while enhaling your breath.stop for few seconds and exhale the breath.Repeat the process from five to ten times.

- Sit on the edge of your seat, and place your feet on the floor. Keep your fingers behind your back. Inhale deeply, move your hands towards the floor and chest upward. Hold your breath for a few seconds and then exhale completely.Again repeat the process

Standing exercise

- Standing straight and bend at the hips to touch your toes. Holding this simple pose for a few seconds is often effective for fighting stress and calming the brain.

- Keep your hands behind your hips, directly behind your back. Raise your crossed hands as high as possible. When lifting, focus on lifting your sternum. Hold the lift for at least 30 seconds, and then let it go. Repeat this movement several times.

Even if you cannot step and spread on the floor, the way you practice yoga, you can get some benefit from doing these movements throughout the day. In many cases, colleagues will not even realize what you are doing when you stretch and soothe the pain to breathe.

Precautions Regarding Yoga

Yoga is taken into account to be very safe, even for older adults or those with disabilities. However, it's still important to be cautious when first getting started.

Although yoga are often customized to satisfy your specific goals and wishes , the National Institutes of Health recommends that anyone with high vital sign, asthma, glaucoma, sciatica and ladies who are pregnant receive clearance from their doctor before beginning.

It's also smart to talk to the yoga teacher about tips for safely modifying or avoiding certain yoga poses which may aggravate your symptoms, especially if you've got a recent injury.

The best thanks to locate a yoga class that's appropriate for you is to ask a trusted source for a recommendation, like your doctor or chiropractor.

Especially if you're new yoga, search for an accredited instructor with certification through a trusted organization just like the Yoga Alliance. The Yoga Alliance requires a minimum of 200 hours of hands-on yoga training. That includes a specified number of required hours in areas including techniques, teaching methodology, anatomy, physiology and philosophy.

Final Thoughts on the Benefits of Yoga

Yoga may be a mind-body practice that has elements of breath control, meditation and therefore the adoption of specific bodily postures (called asanas).

Yoga benefits include reducing pain and improving balance and adaptability . This helps to scale back anxiety, improve sleep and build and maintain muscle mass.

The most popular sorts of yoga practiced within the U.S and Europe are rooted in yoga methods. These include Vinyasa, Ashtanga, Kundalini, Yin, Bikram/hot yoga and Iyengar.

Yoga is typically very safe, even for older adults or those with limitations thanks to injuries, but if you've got high vital sign , asthma, glaucoma, sciatica or are pregnant, it's best to be cautious and get your doctor's clearance first.

Yoga for long life

Yoga can have a profound and positive impact in anti-aging progress i.e yoga fpr long life,some well-known institute studies suggested.

Old age is a natural process of aging.

Ancient techniques for the harmony of the outer and inner body beings through yoga, breath control, meditation, physical movement and gestures… well known to the people of the Western world and parts of Asia.There are reasons for the reported health benefits by reputable institutions. 'Research and supported by health advocates.

To explore the effects of yoga and meditation-based lifestyle interventions (YMLI), randomly assigned to 12 weeks of YMLI on cellular aging in 96 healthy individuals, at the end of the 12-week lesson, the YMLI group expressed many improvements.Both cardinal biomarkers of cellular aging and metabotrophic biomarkers affecting cellular aging compared to baseline values.

The efficacy of the program in the reduced cellular aging process was attributed to activities in ROS and reduced production of pro-inflammatory cytokines and the hormone cortisol, and increased values of telomerase activity in regulated aging progression and reduced hormone end-. To maintain endorphins and homeostasis.

After taking into account the other co-founders, lead author Drs. Madhuri Tolhunesse said, "Lifestyle is an integrated entity, and an intervention like YMLI, which has an overall positive impact on our health, appears to be the most useful versus changing only one aspect.

Other researchers, in a study of yoga breathing in the skin protected against aging, reported the following results

1. Yoga breathing has reduced the psychological aspects of stress and anxiety that have been associated with increasing age

2. Yoga also affected regulated glycation and products (AGE), which have recently been shown to play a role in aging

3. Comprehensive yoga programs that include inhalation and meditation exercises may have profound effects in increased gene expression, including oxidative stress, DNA damage, cell cycle control, aging, and apoptosis.

4. Detoxification

In further analysis, the Dr., Berry-led author stated, "(contracting for general belief) can be translated to improve the interesting correlation of insulin regulation and glucose control and perhaps the accumulation of AGE proteins in body tissues Reversal of Effect on ".

In support of the above differentiation, Dr. at Columbia University College of Physicians and Surgeons. Brown RP launched a yoga breathing investigation into anti-aging progress, suggesting that

1. Yoga breathing (Pranayama) can have a significant and positive effect in bringing the mind to the present moment and reducing stress

2. Yoga delayed the aging process through the expression of victims of breathing depression, anxiety, traumatic stress disorder, and mass disasters.

3. Sadhanas relieve many kinds of suffering.

Finally, after taking other risk factors into consideration, researchers concluded that yoga breathing may affect the longevity mechanism.

Yoga does great for body and soul, especially for more than 60 of us. Here are some examples of vibrant women whose devotion to yoga has paid off in happiness, health and longevity:

Bette Calman, 90, a highly respected yoga teacher for 50 years, she is now "Yoga Super Granny." She gained international fame while acting in an Advil Commercial during the 2016 Super Bowl.

Tao Porchan-Lynch, 98, was recognized as the world's oldest yoga teacher by the Guinness Book of World Records at the age of 93 and is still teaching! His unprecedented background includes twice marching with Mahatma Gandhi and helping people escape the Nazis during World War II as a French resistance fighter. In addition to yoga, he danced ballroom at the "young" age of 85. Tao's mantra is "There is nothing you cannot do." This he has taken to heart all his life and is a great example for all of us.

Ana Pace, age 87, cured her hump posture in just 2 years with the help of a certified back-care yoga instructor. She says she feels amazing now because she can drive and do many things she couldn't do before.

So how does it work? How, in particular, does yoga benefit your body and mind?

In terms of your body, yoga improves balance, which continues to increase as we age. Yoga promotes bone strength, as the nature of the movements themselves improves bone density, which decreases over time.

Yoga is a low-impact form of exercise, which means it gently strengthens your muscles, and in the process, protects them from atrophying. Stronger muscles mean less stress on your joints, thus reducing arthritis.

Yoga also reduces blood pressure without putting undue pressure on your cardiovascular system, which is why it is (for most people, always check with your doctor!) Particularly favorable as part of a low blood pressure-blood pressure program.

Because yoga incorporates deep breathing as a part of practice, more oxygen is circulated throughout the body, for the benefit of your entire internal organs and systems.

Plus side to your mental and emotional state, yoga stimulates some chemical release in the body which can reduce anxiety and promote an overall feeling of relaxation. Because yoga relieves stress, many people find that it improves their sleep.

With that said, yoga has been shown to enhance your memory and ability to process cognitively, something we can all appreciate as we grow in later years!

Why is it important to know about the benefits of yoga? Because it lends itself to a little-known health trick: the more you know how much a thing benefits you, the greater the benefit.

Nowhere did this phenomenon perform better than in the study of notable "hotel maids". Maids in the two hotels did work that lasted more than 30 minutes of daily exercise. At the first hotel, researchers told the maids how many calories they burned through the equivalent of 30 minutes of exercise.

Researchers did not say anything to the maids at the other hotel. After just one month, there was no change in their diet or exercise routine outside of work (which was almost zero), the maids at the first hotel lost an average weight of two pounds, a small percentage of body fat and systolic blood. Average 10 points less pressure.The maids at the other hotel did not change.

What happened? The first hotel maids were now aware of the specific benefits of their work beyond salary. His subconscious transmitted a benefit-message to his body, resulting in weight loss, reduced body fat and lowered blood pressure. Yet the maids were not physically doing anything different.

Of course, maid work is very different from yoga, but the concept is the same. Harness the power of your mind by engaging in the practice of yoga. Know the value and benefits that yoga has for you, both physically and mentally. You can't help but thrive!

Taken as a whole, yoga may have a therapeutic effect in the progression of aging through regulating cellular and psychological manifestations alone or combined with meditation.

Happy and healthy living. Practice Yoga Daily

Yoga is a popular form of exercise that has been known to mankind for more than 5, 000 years. Yoga is a traditional method of meditation, developed in ancient times in India.Most people are aware of the fact that yoga and meditation can help anyone to have some great health benefits.

It is one of the most effective and successful therapy that keep the human body and mind healthy.On a physical level, yoga relieves from many diseases.Practicing different postures gives strength to your body and makes you mentally and physically fit.

Yoga can soak your mind and body properly. If you want to know how Yoga can help you heal yourself, then you need to read the article below carefully. To heal your body you must first start loving yourself.

Now we are going to discuss in detail about how Yoga can help you to heal properly. Make sure you look at the points below carefully.

• Yoga helps you to keep your mind absolutely relaxed and calm. If you want to be relaxed all the time, then yoga can definitely help you a lot. You got to make sure that you make the right choice every time. You should give your body some extra time to heal. You can start by practicing some simple yoga moves and asanas. How can you bring it to the groove?

• The power of acceptance is the strongest ever. You can really benefit a lot from it. You just have to accept your mistakes and strengths as they are. It is useless to be sad at anything. Well, you just have to accept the reality and move on. You can put all your efforts and energy into learning yoga. Tell your trainer about any issues that are bothering you.

• Healing is all about being happy. If you are looking for some enjoyment then you need to practice yoga regularly. You can do anything that makes you happy. You can incorporate yoga into your regular lifestyle. If you are looking for something more fun, you can consider practicing it with your loved ones.

• If you want to take good care of your health then practice caution and mantras. Yoga can help you to cure many disorders including back pain and abdominal pain. You just have to follow the right fitness regime and exercise right.

• The art of letting things go is one of the hardest to learn. It is often said that a person who learns to let things go easily is happiest. So, yoga helps you in this. Regular practice allows you to be healthy easily under all circumstances. You can also learn how to be patient in the most difficult situations.

These are some of the most important things that you should remember about practicing yoga. You need to make sure that if you want to heal your body completely, then you do some yoga yoga regularly. If you are looking for some more information then you can surf the internet. Have lots of fun and have lots of fun.

Today, due to its many benefits, Yoga is one of the leading names in the healthcare and wellness industry, which is why it is important for you to know some more benefits in detail.

Flexibility

Yoga involves the movement and stretch of body parts in many ways. Therefore, it increases flexibility. After a certain period of time, you will be able to gain flexibility in your back, hips and shoulders. However, with age, flexibility naturally decreases which further leads to immobility and pain. Yoga has the ability to modify and postpone this process.

Power

There are many yoga postures that help in weight loss in various ways. The body becomes stronger by giving different poses for a certain period of time.

Muscle tone

Muscle toning is a by-product of yoga. As your body gets stronger, muscle toning increases. Yoga also shapes lean and long muscles.

The balance

A position like standing on one leg helps improve balance. This is one of the most important benefits of doing yoga as we move towards old age.

Pain Relieve

Strength and enhanced flexibility helps in the prevention of back pain, legs or any other part of the body. Nowadays many people complain of back pain due to long working hours on computer. It can also give rise to spinal compression. In such cases, yoga is one of the best treatments without any side effects. It helps in preventing any type of body pain.

Better breathing

Stress is one of the main reasons behind breathing problems. Pranayama is an exercise in yoga that satisfies the problem of breathing. It teaches us how to take deep breaths which purify the entire body system. There are types of breathing styles that help to clear the nasal passages and calm the nervous system. Pranayama is the best exercise for people suffering from allergies.

You can get rid of many diseases by practicing yoga. Yoga is indeed a blessing in disguise for mankind; It is a blessing from the supreme that has no side effects